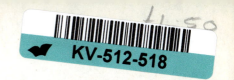

English in Focus: Basic Medical Science

ENGLISH IN FOCUS

English in Basic Medical Science

JOAN MACLEAN

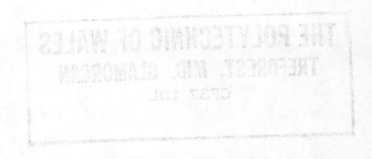
LONDON
OXFORD UNIVERSITY PRESS
1975

Oxford University Press, Ely House, London W.1

GLASGOW NEW YORK TORONTO MELBOURNE WELLINGTON
CAPE TOWN IBADAN NAIROBI DAR ES SALAAM LUSAKA ADDIS ABABA
DELHI BOMBAY CALCUTTA MADRAS KARACHI LAHORE DACCA
KUALA LUMPUR SINGAPORE HONG KONG TOKYO

ISBN 0 19 437515 3   (Student's Book)
ISBN 0 19 437503 x   (Teacher's Edition)

© Oxford University Press 1975

PRINTED AND BOUND IN ENGLAND BY
HAZELL WATSON AND VINEY LTD
AYLESBURY, BUCKS

Contents

Unit 3   Gross Anatomy of the Trunk

Unit 4   Epithelial tissue

Introduction

The aim of this book is to develop knowledge of how English is used for communication in the basic medical sciences. It is intended for students who already know how to handle the common English sentence patterns but who need to learn how these patterns are used in medical writing to convey information and to express medical concepts.

The exercises direct the student's attention to certain features of English which are specific to medical writing. The aim is to provide the student with a strategy for reading more difficult medical texts and to prepare him for making effective use of English in his own writing.

Although the emphasis is on English as a medium of expression in medicine, the basic elements of the language have not been neglected. Pattern practice is provided, particularly in the Use of Language section of each unit, but this kind of work is always presented in relation to a medical context and not simply as an exercise in making sentences for their own sake.

This book does not aim at teaching the subject-matter of medicine, and it does not aim at teaching grammatical structures and vocabulary as such. Its purpose is to show how language is used as a medium for the study of medicine, and so to give students a grounding in one particular set of communication skills in English.

1 The Compartments of the Body

I READING AND COMPREHENSION

[1]The body has three compartments. [2]The first of these consists of active tissue, which is also known as cell mass. [3]This does most of the chemical work of the body.

[4]The second compartment consists of supporting tissue. [5]This is composed of bone minerals, extracellular proteins, and the internal environment, or the extracellular fluid in the blood and lymph.

[6]The third compartment is the energy reserve. [7]This consists of fat, which lies round the principal internal organs and in adipose tissue.

Study the following statements carefully and decide whether they are true or not true according to the information in the reading passage above. Then check your answers by referring to the solutions at the end of the passage.*

(a) The first compartment of the body consists of cell mass.
(b) The second compartment of the body is composed of bone minerals.
(c) The internal environment is composed of the extracellular fluid in the blood and lymph.
(d) The energy reserve is composed of adipose tissue and fat which lies round the principal internal organs.

[8]These compartments cannot be separated by physical dissection, but it is possible to measure them indirectly. [9]This may be done using methods such as the dilution technique.

[10]The size of each compartment varies according to the age, sex and health of the individual. [11]In a healthy young man the total body weight is divided

---

* The following symbols are used in the solutions:

∴   therefore
i.e. that is to say
=   equals, means the same as
≠   does not equal, does not mean the same as

approximately: 55% cell mass, 30% supporting tissue, and 15% energy reserve. [12]A healthy young woman has normally twice as much fat.

(e) The compartments of the body are measurable.
(f) The dilution technique is the only method of measuring the compartments of the body.
(g) The sum of the sizes of the compartments = the total body weight.
(h) The energy reserve of a healthy young woman is approximately 30% of her total body weight.

Solutions

(a) active tissue, which is also known as cell mass (2)
i.e. active tissue = cell mass
     The first compartment of the body consists of active tissue.
∴   *The first compartment of the body consists of cell mass.*

(b) This is composed of bone minerals, extracellular fluid, and the internal environment (5)
     this = the second compartment
     The second compartment of the body is composed of bone minerals AND OTHER THINGS.
∴   It is NOT TRUE that the second compartment of the body is composed of bone minerals (only).

(c) the internal environment, OR the extracellular fluid in the blood and lymph (5)
i.e. the internal environment = the extracellular fluid in the blood and lymph
∴   *The internal environment is composed of the extracellular fluid in the blood and lymph.*

(d) fat, which lies round the principal internal organs and in adipose tissue (7)
=   fat, which lies round the principal internal organs AND fat which lies in adipose tissue
     (adipose tissue is composed of fat and other things)
     The energy reserve is composed of fat, which lies in adipose tissue and round the principal internal organs.
∴   The energy reserve is NOT composed of adipose tissue and fat which lies round the principal internal organs.

(e) it is possible to measure them (8)
=   it is possible to measure the compartments of the body.
∴   *The compartments of the body are measurable.*

(f) methods SUCH AS the dilution technique (9)
= methods LIKE, FOR EXAMPLE, the dilution technique
i.e. The dilution technique is ONE EXAMPLE of the methods of measuring the compartments of the body.
∴ The dilution technique is NOT the only method of measuring the compartments of the body.

(g) the total body weight is divided approximately: 55% cell mass, 30% supporting tissue, and 15% energy reserve (11)
55%+30%+15% = 100%
∴ *The sum of the sizes of the compartments = the total body weight.*

(h) A healthy young woman has normally twice as much fat. (12)
twice as much fat = twice as much energy reserve (see 6, 7)
twice as much energy reserve (as a healthy young man)
= 2×approximately 15% of the total body weight (see 11)
∴ *The energy reserve of a healthy young woman is approximately 30% of her total body weight.*

EXERCISE A *Contextual reference*

Write the following sentences in your notebook, and complete them after studying the reading passage.

EXAMPLE

'This' in sentence 5 refers to the second compartment (OR supporting tissue).

1. 'these' in sentence 2 refers to ......
2. 'this' in sentence 3 refers to ......
3. 'this' in sentence 7 refers to ......

EXERCISE B *Rephrasing*

Rewrite the following sentences, replacing the words printed in italics with expressions from the reading passage which have the same meaning.

EXAMPLE

Fat *is located* round the principal internal organs.
= Fat *lies* round the principal internal organs. (*lies*: from sentence 7)

1. In a healthy young man, approximately 55% of the total body weight consists of *cell mass*.
2. The energy reserve *consists of* fat.
3. The supporting tissue consists partly of the *extracellular fluid in the blood and lymph.*

4. The compartments *are not separable* by physical dissection.
5. Supporting tissue makes up *about* 30% of the total body weight.
6. A young woman has *usually* twice as much fat as a young man.

EXERCISE C *Relationships between statements*

Place the following expressions in the sentences indicated. Where necessary, replace and re-order the words in the sentences, and change the punctuation.

EXAMPLE

however (8)
These compartments cannot be separated by physical dissection. It is, *however*, possible to measure them indirectly.

(a) i.e. (5)

(b) of course (8)

(c) for example (9)

(d) for example (11)

(e) as follows (11)

(f) however (12)

II   USE OF LANGUAGE

EXERCISE A *The description of structure*

1. Copy the following diagram into your notebook. Refer to the reading passage and complete the diagram by filling in the blanks.

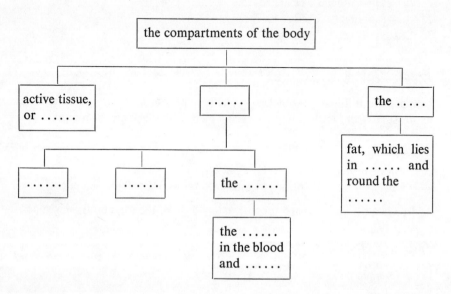

2. Write the following sentences in your notebook, using the completed diagram to finish them. Use the verb *consist of*.

EXAMPLE

The compartments of the body consist of active tissue, or cell mass, supporting tissue, and the energy reserve.

(a) Supporting tissue ......
(b) The energy reserve ......
(c) The internal environment ......

Write the sentences again, this time using the verb *be composed of*.

EXAMPLE

The compartments of the body are composed of active tissue, or cell mass, supporting tissue, and the energy reserve.

3. Write the following sentences in your notebook, using the completed diagram to finish them. Use the verb *form*.

EXAMPLE

Fat, which lies in adipose tissue and round the principal internal organs, forms the energy reserve.

(a) The extracellular fluid in the blood and lymph ......
(b) Active tissue, supporting tissue, and the energy reserve ......
(c) Bone minerals, extracellular proteins, and the internal environment ......

Write the sentences again, this time using the verb *make up*.

EXAMPLE

The fat which lies in adipose tissue and round the principal internal organs makes up the energy reserve.

4. Write the following sentences in your notebook, using the diagram and the verbs *consist of, be composed of, form* and *make up*.
(a) ...... consists of bone minerals, ...
(b) The extracellular fluid in ...... the internal environment.
(c) The energy reserve is ......
(d) Active tissue, ..., and the energy reserve ......
(e) The internal environment consists of ......
(f) Bone minerals, ...

5. Use the following diagrams to write brief descriptions of
(a) the structure of the coraco-acromial arch (1 sentence), and
(b) the structure of skin (3 sentences).

(a)   *The structure of the coraco-acromial arch*

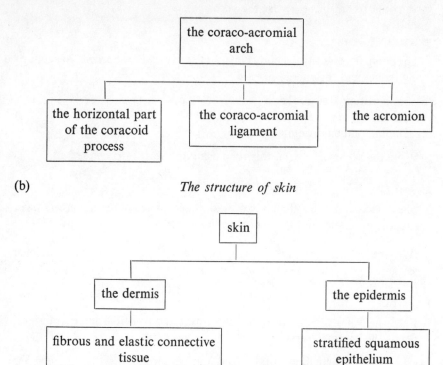

(b)   *The structure of skin*

EXERCISE B *Defining and non-defining relative clauses*

Look at the following sentences:

(a) The large intestine extends from the ileum to the anal canal.
(b) *The large intestine* is about five feet long.
    These two sentences can be combined as follows:
(c) The large intestine, *which* is about five feet long, extends from the ileum to
    the anal canal.

The use of commas with relative clauses

Look at the following sentences:

(d) The inguinal canal, which is an intermuscular slit, lies above the inguinal
    ligament.
(e) Endocrine glands, which secrete into the blood, are found in various parts
    of the body.
(f) Glands which secrete into the blood are known as endocrine glands.
(g) The amount of oxygen which is consumed by the body can be calculated
    using laboratory techniques.

(h) The pleura has a squamous lining, which allows the organs inside to slide over each other.
(i) The pleura has a squamous lining which allows the organs inside to slide over each other.

In sentence (d) and in sentence (e), the relative clause is separated from the rest of the sentence by commas. These relative clauses are called *non-defining* relative clauses. The information in a non-defining relative clause is not essential to the understanding of the rest of the sentence. The non-defining relative clause only adds extra information to the sentence.

In sentence (f) and sentence (g), the relative clause is not separated from the rest of the sentence by commas. The information in the relative clauses is essential to the correct understanding of the rest of the sentence. (Read the sentences again, omitting the relative clauses, and you will see how necessary the relative clauses are.) These are called *defining* relative clauses.

Sometimes a relative clause can be treated either as defining or as non-defining. This depends largely on whether the writer wishes to present the information as essential or additional. Sentence (h) might occur in any paragraph describing the contents of the thorax. Sentence (i) might occur when there is particular emphasis on the *function* of the pleura: i.e. it might follow a description of the mobility of the organs in the thorax.

As a general rule, when a choice can be made between defining and non-defining, the non-defining relative clause, with commas, is the more usual choice in medical writing.

Remember, however, that in sentences like sentences (d), (e), (f), and (g), no choice is possible. The relative clauses in sentences (d) and (e) must be non-defining and must have commas; the relative clauses in sentences (f) and (g) must be defining and must not have commas.

Combine each of the following pairs of sentences into a single sentence. Make the second sentence into a relative clause and insert it into the first sentence in the appropriate place. Use commas when necessary (i.e. when the relative clause is non-defining).

EXAMPLE
    The posterior tibial artery divides into two branches in the foot. The posterior tibial artery runs through the muscle down behind the tibia.
= The posterior tibial artery, which runs through the muscle down behind the tibia, divides into two branches in the foot.

1. The pinna is composed of elastic cartilage covered with skin. The pinna is the part of the ear lying outside the head.
2. Glucose is stored in the body as glycogen. Glycogen is reconverted into glucose when it is needed for energy.
3. The energy reserve is composed of fat. Fat lies round the principal internal organs and in adipose tissue.

4. Valves are found in most veins. Valves direct the blood flow proximally.
5. The bone is called the femur. The bone extends from the hip-bone to the knee.
6. The centre of a tooth consists of pulp. The pulp is surrounded by dentine.
7. The veins of the legs can be divided into two groups, superficial and deep. The two groups, superficial and deep, are joined at intervals by communicating veins.
8. The renal arteries supply the kidneys. The renal arteries arise immediately below the superior mesenteric artery.
9. Ducts and secretory units are surrounded by connective tissue. The connective tissue acts as a supporting framework.
10. Osteoclasts send out processes. The processes erode bone.
11. Synovial membrane secretes a lubricating fluid. Synovial membrane lines joints.
12. Short bones consist of cancellous bone covered with a thin layer of compact bone. Short bones are cuboid in shape.
13. Round the branches of the splenic artery there may be found aggregates of lymphocytes. These aggregates of lymphocytes are known as Malpighian corpuscles.
14. Bile is stored in the gall-bladder. Bile is excreted by the liver.
15. The surface of the body is covered by a layer of skin. A layer of skin protects the body tissues.
16. The fluid makes up the internal environment. The fluid is contained in the blood and lymph.
17. One compartment of the body is active tissue. Active tissue is also known as cell mass.
18. The lacrimal gland is continually secreting fluid. The fluid keeps the eye moist and free from dust particles.

EXERCISE C *Relative clauses with prepositions*

In medical writing there are many relative clauses with a preposition before *which*. Such clauses are formed in the following way:

(a) Connective tissue is a matrix.
(b) More highly organized tissues are embedded *in this matrix*.
= Connective tissue is a matrix *in which* more highly organized tissues are embedded.

Combine each of the following pairs of sentences into a single sentence containing a relative clause beginning with a preposition + *which*. Use commas when the clause is a non-defining one.

1. The cerebellum is the centre for reflexes. Muscles are co-ordinated and balance is maintained by these reflexes.
2. The ear has a central part, the vestibule. From the vestibule three canals and the cochlea are given off.

3. The muscle is known as the mylo-hyoid. The hyoid bone is connected to the mandible by the muscle.
4. There are little branching tubes in dentine. Nutritive material is conveyed from the bloodstream through the little branching tubes in dentine.
5. The cranium is a large, bony case. The brain is protected by this large, bony case.
6. In the epidermis there are different strata. In the different strata, the cells have distinctive anatomical features.
7. Strands of Schwann cells provide surfaces. The growing axons cling to these surfaces.
8. The stomach is attached to the abdominal wall by its mesentery. Through its mesentery run blood vessels, lymphatics and nerves.
9. Some motor fibres enter the medulla oblongata. They form two pyramidal tracts in the medulla oblongata.
10. Endocrine glands have lost their connection with the alimentary cavity. They were derived from the alimentary cavity.
11. The pre-vertebral fascia provides a foundation. The pharynx and the oesophagus can slide upon this foundation.
12. The bone is pierced by many openings, or foramina. The vessels and nerves pass through the openings, or foramina.
13. There are small veins in the palms and fingers. The superficial and deep palmar arches are formed from the small veins in the palms and fingers.
14. The capsule of a lymph node is made up of fibrous tissue. There is a certain amount of plain muscle in the fibrous tissue.
15. The walls of the capillary and the alveolus fuse to make a very thin wall. The interchange of gases takes place through this very thin wall.

III INFORMATION TRANSFER

Study the following illustrations and the paragraphs beneath them. Write the paragraphs in your notebook and complete them with reference to the illustrations.

1.

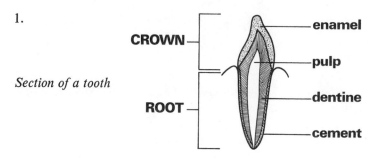

Section of a tooth

A tooth consists of two main parts: a ...... and a ......
...... makes up the centre of the tooth.
This is surrounded by ......
In the crown, the dentine is covered with ......
In the ......, the dentine ......

2.

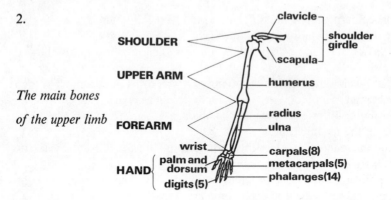

The main bones

of the upper limb

The upper limb ...... the shoulder, the upper ......, ..., and the hand.
The shoulder girdle is made up of the ...... and the ......
The bone of the upper arm is known as the ......
The bones of the ...... consist of the .... and the ....
The hand may be divided into two parts: the ...... and ......, and the
five ...... Fourteen ...... make ...... the bones of the five ......,
five metacarpal bones support the ......, and eight ...... form ......

3.

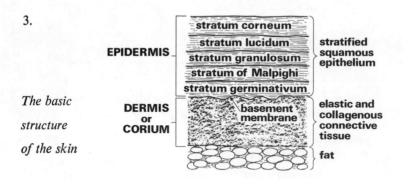

The basic

structure

of the skin

The ...... is composed ...... main layers. The superficial layer is known
as the ......; the deeper ......
The epidermis ...... stratified ...... Cells are produced in its deepest layer,
the stratum ......, and become flatter as they are pushed up to the surface
layer, or stratum ......

The dermis ...... elastic ...... The elastic tissue predominates in super-ficial levels, where it ...... a basement ...... which acts as a foundation for the ......

Below the dermis is a ...... of subcutaneous ......

IV GUIDED WRITING

STAGE 1 *Sentence building*

Join each of the groups of sentences below into one long sentence, using the additional words printed in capital letters above each group. Omit words printed in italics and put relative clauses in the places marked by dots. Make whatever changes you think are necessary in the punctuation of the sentences.

EXAMPLE

WHICH

The weighing machine ...... is one of the doctor's most useful tools.
The weighing machine can be found in any clinic.
It is used for assessing the general health of his patients.

= The weighing machine which can be found in any clinic is one of the doctor's most useful tools for assessing the general health of his patients.

1. WHICH
Oedema ...... is a typical feature of many cardiac, renal and liver diseases.
Oedema is due to an increase in the extracellular water.

2. WITH/AND
The body is composed of different compartments.
Each *compartment has* a different function.
These compartments are affected differently by different diseases.

3. THAT
It must always be kept in mind.
The body is not a uniform mass.

4. IF/THEN
The size of the increase in the supporting tissue equals the size of the reduction in the other two compartments.
The total body weight remains constant.

5. TOO/A/TO BE
   The weighing machine is *a* crude tool.
   It cannot be an accurate guide to health.

6. AND/BUT/WHICH
   There is a reduction in the cell mass.
   There is a reduction in the energy reserve.
   There is an increase in the supporting tissue ....
   This increase is caused by oedema.

STAGE 2 *Paragraph building*

Add the following material to the sentences indicated:

write 'for example' at the beginning of sentence 1
write 'it' instead of 'the body' in sentence 2
add 'however' to sentence 3
add 'in cases like these' to the beginning of sentence 5
write 'in wasting diseases too,' at the beginning of sentence 6.

Rewrite the six sentences in a logical order to make a paragraph, and include the example as the first sentence of the paragraph.

When you have written your paragraph, re-read it and make sure the sentences are presented in a logical order. Give the paragraph a suitable title. Compare your paragraph with the relevant paragraph in the Free Reading section (p. 13). Make any changes that you think are necessary, but remember that sentences can often be arranged in more than one way.

STAGE 3 *Paragraph reconstruction*

Read through the paragraph again. Make sure you know all the words, using a dictionary if necessary. Without referring to your previous work, rewrite the paragraph. Here are some notes to help you.

weighing machine – useful tool – general health
keep in mind – body – not uniform mass
different compartments – different function – affected differently – different
   diseases
oedema – increase in extracellular water – typical feature – cardiac, renal
   and liver diseases
wasting diseases – less cell mass – less energy reserve – more supporting
   tissue – oedema
if increase = reduction – total body weight – constant
weighing machine – too crude

V FREE READING

Read the following passage in your own time. Try to find additional examples of the points you have studied in this unit.

The Measurement of the Compartments of the Body

The weighing machine which can be found in any clinic is one of the doctor's most useful tools for assessing the general health of his patients. It must always be kept in mind, however, that the body is not a uniform mass. It is composed of different compartments, each with a different function, and these compartments are affected differently by different diseases. For example, oedema, which is due to an increase in the extracellular water, is a typical feature of many cardiac, renal and liver diseases. In wasting diseases too, there is a reduction in the cell mass and in the energy reserve, but there is an increase in the supporting tissue, which is caused by oedema. If the size of the increase in the supporting tissue equals the size of the reduction in the other two compartments, then the total body weight remains constant. In cases like these, the weighing machine is too crude a tool to be an accurate guide to health.

The different compartments of the body can be measured separately, but complicated laboratory and clinical procedures are necessary. The approximate size of the cell mass may be calculated from the size of the cell water, which is obtained from the difference between the total body water and the extracellular water. The size of the total body water may be measured by the dilution technique, using substances such as deuterium oxide and ethyl alcohol. These may be administered orally or by intravenous injection. The size of the extracellular water may be measured by injecting into the body substances such as sodium thiocyanate. The energy reserve can be determined by measurements of body density. The weight of the bone minerals and the extracellular proteins can be calculated only by finding the difference between the total body weight and all other parts.

Measurement of the compartments of the body by these procedures has provided new insight into how the body works in health and in disease. The procedures are too complicated, however, for use in normal clinical practice.

2 Sources of Energy

I READING AND COMPREHENSION

[1]The fuels of the body are carbohydrates, fats and proteins. [2]These are taken in the diet. [3]They are found mainly in cereal grains, vegetable oils, meat, fish, and dairy products.

[4]Carbohydrates are the principal source of energy in most diets. [5]They are absorbed into the bloodstream in the form of glucose. [6]Glucose not needed for immediate use is converted into glycogen and stored in the liver. [7]When the blood sugar concentration goes down, the liver reconverts some of its stored glycogen into glucose.

[8]Fats make up the second largest source of energy in most diets. [9]They are stored in adipose tissue and round the principal internal organs. [10]If excess carbohydrate is taken in, this can be converted into fat and stored. [11]The stored fat is utilized when the liver is empty of glycogen.

(a) The fuels of the body are taken in the diet.
(b) Carbohydrates, fats and proteins are found only in cereal grains, vegetable oils, meat, fish and dairy products.
(c) Carbohydrates are stored in the liver as glycogen.
(d) Fats are stored only round the principal internal organs.

[12]Proteins are essential for the growth and rebuilding of tissue, but they can also be utilized as a source of energy. [13]In some diets, such as the diet of the Eskimo, they form the main source of energy. [14]Proteins are first broken down into amino acids. [15]Then they are absorbed into the blood and pass round the body. [16]Amino acids not used by the body are eventually excreted in the urine in the form of urea. [17] Proteins, unlike carbohydrates and fats, cannot be stored for future use.

(e) Proteins are essential for growth and energy.
(f) Proteins are the main source of energy in most diets.

(g) Amino acids which are not absorbed into the blood are excreted in the urine in the form of urea.

(h) Carbohydrates and fats cannot be stored for future use.

Solutions

(a) These are taken in the diet. (2)
  these = carbohydrates, fats and proteins = the fuels of the body (1)
∴ *The fuels of the body are taken in the diet.*

(b) They (carbohydrates, fats and proteins) are found MAINLY in cereal grains, vegetable oils, meat, fish, and dairy products. (3)
  mainly ≠ only
∴ It is NOT TRUE that carbohydrates, fats and proteins are found ONLY in cereal grains, vegetable oils, meat, fish and dairy products.

(c) They (carbohydrates) are absorbed into the bloodstream in the form of glucose. (5)
i.e. Carbohydrates are converted into glucose.
  Glucose not needed for immediate use is converted into glycogen and stored in the liver. (6)
i.e. Glucose is stored in the liver as glycogen.
∴ *Carbohydrates are stored in the liver as glycogen.*

(d) They (fats) are stored in adipose tissue and round the principal internal organs. (9)
i.e. Fats are stored round the principal internal organs AND ALSO in adipose tissue.
∴ It is NOT TRUE that fats are stored ONLY round the principal internal organs.

(e) Proteins are essential for the growth and rebuilding of tissue. (12)
i.e. Proteins are essential for growth.
  they (proteins) CAN also be utilized as a source of energy. (12)
  can ≠ must
i.e. Proteins are not essential for energy.
∴ Proteins are essential for growth but they are not essential for energy.
∴ Proteins are NOT essential for growth AND energy.

(f) In SOME diets, such as the diet of the Eskimo, they (proteins) form the main source of energy. (13)
  in some diets ≠ in most diets
∴ Proteins are NOT the main source of energy in MOST diets.

(g) They (amino acids) are absorbed into the blood. (15)
Amino acids not used by the body are eventually excreted in the urine in the form of urea. (16)
but All amino acids are absorbed into the blood in the first place. (see 15)
∴   It is NOT TRUE that amino acids which are not absorbed into the blood are excreted in the urine in the form of urea.

(h) Proteins, unlike carbohydrates and fats, cannot be stored for future use. (17)
i.e. Carbohydrates and fats are not like proteins.
Proteins CANNOT be stored for future use.
∴   Carbohydrates and fats CAN be stored for future use.

EXERCISE A *Contextual reference*

Write the following sentences in your notebook and complete them after studying the reading passage.

1. 'these' in sentence 2 refers to .. ....
2. 'they' in sentence 5 refers to ......
3. 'this' in sentence 10 refers to ......
4. 'they' in sentence 13 refers to ......
5. 'they' in sentence 15 refers to ......

EXERCISE B *Rephrasing*

Rewrite the following sentences replacing the words printed in italics with expressions from the reading passage which have the same meaning.

1. Cereal grains are one of the *main* sources of carbohydrate in the diet.
2. Glucose *which is not needed immediately* is converted into glycogen.
3. Carbohydrates are stored in the liver *as* glycogen.
4. The liver reconverts some of its glycogen when the blood sugar concentration *falls*.
5. If *too much* sugar is *ingested*, it is excreted in the urine.
6. A well-balanced diet is *necessary* for growth and energy.
7. *In contrast with* milk, beef contains no vitamin A and no vitamin C.
8. Glycogen, derived from glucose, is stored *for later use*.

EXERCISE C *Relationships between statements*

Place the following expressions in the sentences indicated. Where necessary, replace and re-order the words in the sentences, and change the punctuation.

(a) of course (4)   (d) indeed (13)
(b) also (9)   (e) for example (13)
(c) in addition (12)   (f) therefore (17)

II USE OF LANGUAGE

EXERCISE A absorb, store, convert

1. Copy the following diagram into your notebook. Refer to the reading passage and complete the diagram by filling in the blanks.

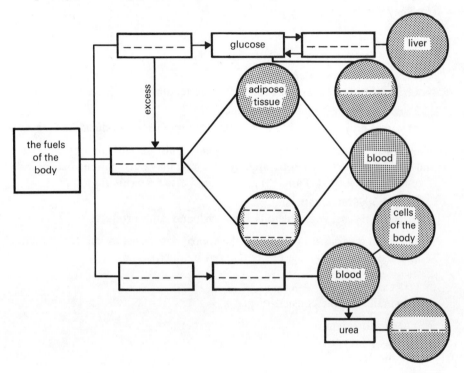

2. Write the following sentences in your notebook, using the completed diagram to finish them. Use the verbs *absorb*, *convert* and *store*.
   N.B. The verbs are all used here in the passive.

   (a) Carbohydrates ... into glucose.
   (b) Glucose ... into glycogen.
   (c) Glucose ... into the blood.
   (d) Glycogen ... in the liver.
   (e) Glycogen ... back into glucose, and this ... into the blood.
   (f) Fats ... in ... and round the ...
   (g) Proteins ... into ...
   (h) Amino acids ... into the blood.
   (i) The amino acids not needed by the cells of the body ... into urea and excreted in the ...

EXERCISE B *Listing* (i)

1. Write out the following lists in your notebook, completing them with reference to the first paragraph of the reading passage.

(a) The fuels of the body are 1. ......
2. ......
3. ......

(b) They are found mainly in 1. ......
2. ......
3. ......
4. ......
5. ......

Notice how these lists are punctuated in the reading passage:

(a) carbohydrates, fats and proteins
(b) cereal grains, vegetable oils, meat, fish, and dairy products

When a list is written out within a sentence, items are separated by commas and the last two items are separated by *and*. You may put a comma before *and* if you want to. Lists (a) and (b) above could also be written:

(a) carbohydrates, fats, and proteins
(b) cereal grains, vegetable oils, meat, fish and dairy products

2. Write out the following lists with the appropriate punctuation. Insert them into the sentences at the places marked by dots.

EXAMPLE
The small intestine consists of ...

1. the duodenum
2. the jejunum
3. the ileum

The small intestine consists of the duodenum, the jejunum, and the ileum. (*or*: The small intestine consists of the duodenum, the jejunum and the ileum.)

(a) The spleen touches ...
1. the diaphragm
2. the end of the pancreas
3. the left kidney

(b) The principal bones of the face are ...
1. the frontal bone
2. the temporal bone
3. the nasal bone
4. the maxilla
5. the mandible

(c) The ... enter the lungs on their inner side.
    1. bronchi
    2. blood vessels
    3. lymphatic vessels
    4. nerves

(d) The following are the chief branches of the aorta: ...
    1. the coeliac artery
    2. the superior mesenteric artery
    3. the renal arteries
    4. the gonadal arteries
    5. the inferior mesenteric artery

(e) Splenic pulp consists of a network of fibrous connective tissue with ... in the meshes.
    1. red blood corpuscles
    2. lymphocytes
    3. reticulo-endothelial cells

(f) The functions of the back muscles are ...
    1. to support the spine
    2. to move the spine
    3. to move the extremities of the body

EXERCISE C *Short-form relative clauses* (i)

A relative clause containing a *passive* verb can be shortened as follows:

(a) Glycogen *which has been stored in the liver* can be reconverted into glucose.
(b) Glycogen *stored in the liver* can be reconverted into glucose.

A relative clause containing an *active* verb can be shortened as follows:

(c) Mucous membrane lines spaces *which communicate with the outside of the body*.
(d) Mucous membrane lines spaces *communicating with the outside of the body*.

    Rewrite the relative clauses in the following sentences as in examples (b) or (d) above.

    N.B. Retain the commas when the clause is non-defining.

    1. Iron, which is found mainly in meat, eggs, beans and peas, is an essential part of the diet.

2. The acidity of chyme in the duodenum is reduced by bile, a substance which is produced by the liver.
3. The cells which form the islets of Langerhans have no ducts.
4. The oesophagus is a tube which leads from the pharynx to the stomach.
5. The envelope which encloses haemoglobin is a semi-permeable membrane.
6. Fat which has been absorbed into the lacteals passes into the bloodstream at the left internal jugular vein.
7. The matrix of bone is made up of an inorganic material, which contains calcium phosphate.
8. The mandible is made up of two halves, which fuse at the midline to form the chin.
9. Most of the energy which is required by the body is derived from carbohydrates and fats.
10. The intestine receives food which is already partly digested.
11. The cytoplasm of a neutrophil contains numerous granules which stain with acid and basic dyes.
12. Pepsin and hydrochloric acid are among constituents of the juice which is secreted by the stomach.
13. The epithelium which lines the urinary passages is referred to as transitional epithelium.
14. Bulk in the faeces may be provided by cellulose, which is taken in the diet.
15. Reticular tissue is a special type of areolar tissue, which consists of a loose network of fine collagen fibres.

EXERCISE D *Short-form relative clauses* (ii)

Rewrite the following sentences so that each contains a relative clause beginning with *which*. Take care in choosing active or passive voice.

1. The shaft of a long bone consists of compact bone surrounding a tubular cavity.
2. Glycogen, derived from glucose, is stored for future use.
3. Food broken down by enzymes is absorbed through the lining of the intestine into the blood.
4. Amino acids not required for new protoplasm can be utilized by the liver in the manufacture of fibrinogen.
5. The pyloric sphincter, separating the stomach from the duodenum, opens periodically to allow some of the chyme to pass through.
6. Vitamin K is required for the formation of prothrombin, a substance needed for blood-clotting.
7. The spinal cord gives off paired spinal nerves, passing out between the vertebrae.
8. Glucose taken out of the bloodstream by the muscles is converted into glycogen until needed.

9. Juices secreted by the stomach, liver and pancreas all play a part in the digestive process.
10. The epithelial cells forming the mucous membrane of the stomach are columnar in shape.
11. The thyroid gland is an endocrine gland consisting of two lobes joined at their lower ends.
12. The portal vein carries to the liver the products of digestion absorbed into the bloodstream.
13. Air is expelled from the thorax as a result of a passive elastic recoil occurring in the lungs and the thoracic wall.
14. The small intestine receives sucrose broken down into glucose and fructose.
15. There are muscles at the base of the little finger forming the hypothenar eminence.

EXERCISE E *Short-form relative clauses* (iii)

Complete the following sentences so that each contains a short-form relative clause. Use the *-ing* or the *-ed* form of the verbs below.

attach	cover	separate	form
grow	produce	lie	contain

1. The marrow cells ... within bone have a haemopoietic function.
2. The serous membrane ... the pericardium is reflected over the surface of the heart.
3. The diaphragm is a dome-shaped muscle ... to the ribs and vertebrae.
4. The skull may be divided into the face, with its sinuses and cavities, and the cranium, ... the brain.
5. Calcified cartilage and dead cells are replaced by ... bone.
6. The mediastinum is a partition ... the two lungs.
7. The movements of the vertebral column are produced by muscles widely ... from each other.
8. The bones ... the hand and wrist are the carpals, metacarpals and phalanges.
9. A mucous membrane ... with columnar ciliated epithelium lines the nasal cavities.
10. The infratemporal fossa is a space ... beneath the base of the skull between the pharynx and the mandible.
11. Ovulation is suppressed by progesterone, a hormone ... by the corpus luteum.
12. Sweat glands are tubes of epithelium, ... down from the epidermis into the corium.

III   INFORMATION TRANSFER

The percentage of daily requirements in beef, haddock and milk

1. Study the following graph and the paragraph beneath it. Write the paragraph in your notebook and complete it with reference to the graph.

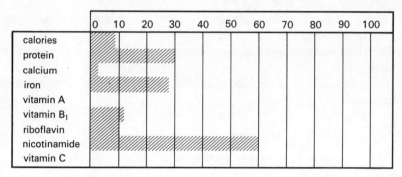

Percentage of daily requirements in 4 ounces of beef

Four ounces of beef supply 60% of the daily requirement of ......,
...... % of the protein and about 28% ...... Beef contains no ...... and
no ......, and only ...... 3% of the necessary ......

2. Compare the following graph with the paragraph above, and complete the paragraph beneath it. Write the paragraph in your notebook.

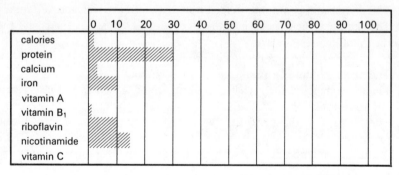

Percentage of daily requirements in 4 ounces of haddock

...... and four ounces of beef supply almost equal amounts of ......,
...... and ...... Like ......, haddock contains no ...... and no ......,
but haddock supplies less vitamin ...... beef. Beef is a greater source of
......, ... and ...... It has about 45% more nicotinamide, ...
more iron, and ...... than haddock.

3. Use the following graph to write a paragraph describing the percentage of daily requirements contained in a half pint of milk. (3-4 sentences)

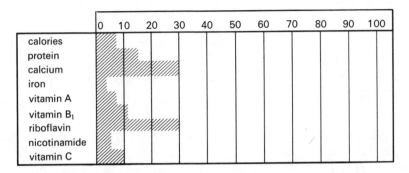

Percentage of daily requirements in a half pint of milk

4. Compare the graph in 1 with the graph in 3. Write a paragraph describing the differences between beef and milk as sources of daily requirements. (4-5 sentences)

IV GUIDED WRITING

STAGE 1 *Sentence building*

Join each of the groups of sentences below into one longer sentence, using the additional words printed in capital letters above some of the groups. Omit words in italics. You may use relative clauses or short-form relative clauses, but note that these are NOT indicated.

1. The most powerful enzyme is pepsin.
   Pepsin begins the process of converting proteins into amino acids.
2. BOTH/AND
   The stomach has a chemical *function*.
   The stomach has a physical function.
3. Waves of peristalsis churn the food particles into a semi-solid mass.
   The semi-solid mass is known as chyme.
4. ALTHOUGH/UNTIL
   Enzymatic action begins in the mouth.
   The major processes of digestion do not occur *in the mouth*.
   The food passes down through the oesophagus into the stomach.
5. Waves of contraction and relaxation *occur*.
   These waves are known as peristalsis.
   They sweep the walls of the stomach.
6. The walls of the stomach secrete gastric juices.

The gastric juices are composed of several enzymes and hydrochloric acid. *The walls of the stomach* are protected by a layer of mucus.

STAGE 2 *Paragraph building*

Rewrite the six sentences in a logical order to make a paragraph, making the following changes to the sentences indicated:

write 'they' instead of 'waves of peristalsis' in sentence 3
write 'in addition, during these chemical reactions' at the beginning of sentence 5.

When you have written your paragraph, re-read it and make sure the sentences are presented in a logical order. Give the paragraph a suitable title. Compare your paragraph with the relevant paragraph in the Free Reading passage. Make any changes that you think are necessary, but remember that sentences can often be arranged in more than one way.

STAGE 3 *Paragraph reconstruction*

Read through the paragraph again. Make sure you know all the words, using a dictionary if necessary. Without referring to your previous work, rewrite the paragraph. Here are some notes to help you.

enzymatic action – mouth – major digestive processes – stomach
stomach – two functions – (1) chemical (2) physical
(1) walls – protected by mucus – secrete gastric juices – several enzymes – hydrochloric acid
most powerful – pepsin – begins process – converting proteins – amino acids
(2) waves of contraction and relaxation – peristalsis – sweep walls of stomach
churn food particles – semi-solid mass – chyme.

V FREE READING

Read the following passage in your own time. Try to find additional examples of the points you have studied in this and other units.

The Process of Digestion

The process of digestion begins when food is taken into the mouth. Chewing breaks the food into smaller pieces, thereby exposing more surfaces to the saliva. Saliva itself has a double function. It moistens the food, so facilitating swallowing, and it contains ptyalin, which begins the conversion of starch into simple sugars.

Although enzymatic action begins in the mouth, the major processes of digestion do not occur until the food passes down through the oesophagus into the stomach. The stomach has both a chemical and a physical function. The walls of the stomach, which are protected by a layer of mucus, secrete gastric juices composed of several enzymes and hydrochloric acid. The most powerful enzyme is pepsin, which begins the process of converting proteins into amino acids. In addition, during these chemical reactions waves of contraction and relaxation, known as peristalsis, sweep the walls of the stomach. They churn the food particles into a semi-solid mass known as chyme.

From the stomach, the chyme passes into the small intestine through the pyloric sphincter. Much undigested material is still present. Proteins have not been completely broken down, starches are still being converted into simple sugars, and fats remain in large globules. In the small intestine the process of digestion is completed by the action of bile, which is secreted by the liver and released by the gall bladder, and by the action of various enzymes, such as lipase and diastase, which are secreted by the pancreas, and erepsin and invertase, secreted by the walls of the small intestine. Foods which are still undigested pass on in a liquid state into the large intestine, and are now called faeces.

Absorption of the products of digestion takes place mainly through the wall of the small intestine. Its inner surface is covered with minute hair-like projections called villi. Each villus contains several blood capillaries and a specialized lymphatic vessel, known as a lacteal. Glucose, fructose, galactose and the amino acids are all absorbed directly into the blood by entering the blood capillaries inside the villi. Glycerol and the fatty acids, on the other hand, pass into the lacteals. The lymph then carries the fat up to the left internal jugular vein, where it enters the bloodstream.

3 Gross Anatomy of the Trunk

I READING AND COMPREHENSION

---

¹The trunk is the central part of the body. ²The neck and head extend above the trunk and are continuous with it. ³The upper limbs are attached to either side of the trunk and the lower limbs extend downwards from it. ⁴The outer tissues of the trunk form the body wall.

⁵The trunk consists of two main cavities, namely the thorax and the abdomen. ⁶These are separated by a dome-shaped muscle known as the diaphragm. ⁷The thorax lies above the diaphragm, and the abdomen lies below it.

⁸The posterior wall of both cavities is composed of the vertebral column and its related muscles.

(a)   the trunk = the body
(b)   The neck and head form part of the trunk.
(c)   The abdomen is bounded superiorly by the diaphragm.
(d)   The abdomen is bounded posteriorly by the vertebral column and its related muscles.

⁹The thoracic cavity is bounded at the sides and front by the ribs, the sternum, and the intercostal muscles. ¹⁰The principal internal organs contained in the thorax are the heart and the lungs.

¹¹The abdomen is the largest cavity in the body. ¹²It consists of two parts: the abdominal cavity proper and the pelvic cavity.

(e)   The walls of the thoracic cavity are composed of the ribs, the sternum, and the intercostal muscles.
(f)   The heart and the lungs lie within the thoracic cavity.
(g)   The cavity above the diaphragm is larger than the cavity below the diaphragm.
(h)   The abdominal cavity is part of the abdominal cavity proper.
(i)   The pelvic cavity can be said to be part of the abdomen.

[13]The lateral and anterior walls of the abdominal cavity proper are formed mainly by three layers of muscle which run concentrically round the cavity. [14]The organs of digestion are the principal internal organs contained in the abdomen.

[15]The pelvic cavity, or pelvis, lies below the abdominal cavity and is continuous with it. [16]It is bounded anteriorly and laterally by bone. [17]The contents of the pelvis are the urinary bladder, the lower part of the large intestine, the rectum, and some of the reproductive organs.

(j) The organs of digestion are the only internal organs contained in the abdomen.
(k) The abdominal cavity and the pelvic cavity are separated by layers of muscle.
(l) The reproductive organs are found in the pelvis.

Solutions

(a) The trunk is the central part of the body. (1)
i.e. The trunk is part of the body.
 ∴ It is NOT TRUE that the trunk = the body.

(b) The neck and head extend ABOVE the trunk. (2)
 ∴ The neck and head do NOT form part of the trunk.

(c) These (the thorax and the abdomen) are separated by ... the diaphragm. (6)
i.e. The abdomen is bounded by the diaphragm.
 The abdomen lies below it (the diaphragm). (7)
 ∴ *The abdomen is bounded superiorly by the diaphragm.*

(d) The posterior wall of both cavities (the thorax and the abdomen) is composed of the vertebral column and its related muscles. (8)
 ∴ The posterior wall of the abdomen is composed of the vertebral column and its related muscles.
i.e. *The abdomen is bounded posteriorly by the vertebral column and its related muscles.*

(e) The thoracic cavity is bounded at the sides and front by the ribs, the sternum, and the intercostal muscles. (9)
i.e. The lateral and anterior walls (but NOT the posterior wall) are composed of the ribs, the sternum, and the intercostal muscles.
 ∴ It is NOT TRUE that (all) the walls of the thoracic cavity are composed of the ribs, the sternum and the intercostal muscles.

(f)   The principal internal organs contained in the thorax are the heart and the lungs. (10)

i.e.   The heart and the lungs are contained in the thorax.

∴   *The heart and the lungs lie within the thoracic cavity.*

(g)   The abdomen is the largest cavity in the body. (11)
       The abdomen is the cavity below the diaphragm. (7)

i.e.   The cavity below the diaphragm is the largest cavity in the body.

∴   The cavity above the diaphragm is NOT larger than the cavity below the diaphragm.

(h)   It (the abdomen = (here) the abdominal cavity) consists of two parts: the abdominal cavity proper and the pelvic cavity. (12)

i.e.   the abdominal cavity = the abdominal cavity proper + the pelvic cavity

∴   It is NOT TRUE that the abdominal cavity is part of the abdominal cavity proper.

(i)   It (the abdomen) consists of two parts: the abdominal cavity proper and the pelvic cavity. (12)

i.e.   The abdominal cavity proper and the pelvic cavity are two parts of the abdomen.

∴   *The pelvic cavity can be said to be part of the abdomen.*

(j)   The organs of digestion are the PRINCIPAL internal organs contained in the abdomen. (14)

∴   The organs of digestion are NOT the ONLY internal organs contained in the abdomen.

(k)   The pelvic cavity ... is continuous with it (the abdominal cavity). (15)

i.e.   Nothing separates the abdominal cavity and the pelvic cavity.

∴   The abdominal cavity and the pelvic cavity are NOT separated by layers of muscle.

(l)   The contents of the pelvis are ... some of the reproductive organs. (17)

i.e.   SOME of the reproductive organs are found in the pelvis.

∴   It is NOT TRUE that (all) the reproductive organs are found in the pelvis.

EXERCISE A *Contextual reference*

Write the following sentences in your notebook and complete them after studying the reading passage.

1. 'it' in sentence 2 refers to ......
2. 'these' in sentence 6 refers to ......
3. 'it' in sentence 7 refers to ......

4. 'its' in sentence 8 refers to ......
5. 'it' in sentence 15 refers to ......
6. 'it' in sentence 16 refers to ......

EXERCISE B *Rephrasing*

Rewrite the following sentences, replacing the words printed in italics with expressions from the reading passage which have the same meaning.
1. The body wall *is composed of* the outer tissues of the trunk.
2. The muscle which separates the thorax from the abdomen is *referred to as* the diaphragm.
3. The vertebral column and its *associated* muscles form the posterior wall of the thorax.
4. The abdomen *is situated* below the diaphragm.
5. The *organs contained within* the abdomen are *principally* the organs of digestion.
6. The *pelvic cavity* lies *inferior to* the *abdominal cavity*.
7. The pelvis is bounded *laterally and anteriorly* by bone.
8. Some of the *organs of reproduction* are found in the pelvis.

EXERCISE C *Analysis into lists*

The reading passage contains several lists. Write out the following lists in your notebook, completing them with reference to the reading passage.

1. The trunk contains two main cavities:
   1. ......
   2. ......
2. The posterior wall of both cavities is composed of:
   1. ......
   2. ......
3. The thorax is bounded at the sides and front by:
   1. ......
   2. ......
   3. ......
4. The principal organs in the thorax are:
   1. ......
   2. ......
5. The abdomen consists of two parts:
   1. ......
   2. ......
6. The contents of the pelvis are:
   1. ......
   2. ......
   3. ......
   4. ......

II USE OF LANGUAGE

EXERCISE A *The anatomical position*

Read the following passage, paying special attention to the anatomical terms.

The Anatomical Position

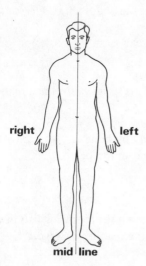

In the anatomical position the body is upright. The arms are by the sides and the legs are parallel to each other. The palms of the hands, the feet, the face and the eyes are all directed forwards.

The anatomical position is the basis of all descriptions of the position of structures in the body. For example, the head is always said to be *above* the feet, even when the patient is lying down.

Descriptions may relate directly to the anatomical position:

EXAMPLES

The trunk is the *central* part of the body.
The legs extend *downwards*.

Descriptions may be made with reference to other structures:

EXAMPLES

The abdomen is *below the thorax*.
The diaphragm lies *between the abdomen and the thorax*.

Special terms are used to describe sections made through the body. A *median* section is made vertically through the midline and cuts the body into two halves, right and left. A *sagittal* section is any section which is parallel to the median section. A *coronal* section is also a vertical section, but it is made from side to side. A horizontal section is often known as a *transverse* section or a *cross-section*. A section may be *oblique* or at any other angle, e.g. the section of a tooth on p. 9 is longitudinal, and the section of skin on p. 10 is made at right angles to the surface.

EXAMPLES

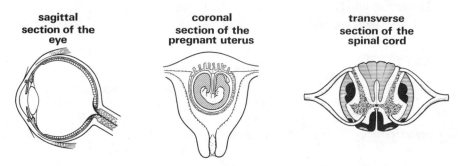

| sagittal section of the eye | coronal section of the pregnant uterus | transverse section of the spinal cord |

EXERCISE B *Locative adjectives*

The following locative adjectives are in common use in medical writing. *Locative* means *describing situation or place*.
(a) right, left
(b) inner, outer
(c) upper, lower
(d) internal, external (especially of hollow structures)
(e) superficial, deep (= nearer and farther from the surface of the body)
(f) central, peripheral (= nearer and farther from the centre of the body)
(g) proximal, distal (especially of limbs; = nearer and farther from the trunk)
(h) superior, inferior (= higher and lower, in transverse planes)
(i) anterior, posterior (= nearer the front, nearer the back, in coronal planes)
(j) medial, lateral (= nearer and farther from the midline, in sagittal planes)

Notice that the adjectives (e) – (j) may be used as follows:

the *superior* vena cava
The head is *superior to* the heart.
the *lateral* surface of the lung
The lungs lie *lateral to* the heart.

Choose adjectives from the list above to complete the following sentences. Write the sentences in your notebook.
1. The head is ... to the feet.
2. The sternum is ... to the heart.
3. The left lung lies ... to the heart.
4. The humerus articulates at its ... end with the radius and ulna.
5. The ulna is ... to the radius.
6. The stomach is situated ... to the heart.
7. The thorax is bordered on the ... region by the vertebral column and its associated muscles.
8. The phalanges are found at the ... ends of the limbs.
9. The pelvic cavity is ... to the abdominal cavity.

10. ... to the dermis lies a layer of subcutaneous fat.
11. The thumb is on the ... side of the hand.
12. The right lung lies ... to the heart.

EXERCISE C *Locative verbs*

The position of structures in the body may be described according to:
 (i) *position*: The stomach lies in the abdominal cavity.
          The oesophagus is posterior to the trachea.
(ii) *direction*: The stomach extends downwards and to the left.
          The oesophagus descends through the thorax.
The table below shows some common verbs of position and direction.

TABLE 1

position	direction
be	be directed
be found	lead
lie	run
be situated	extend
be located	pass
	descend
	ascend

Adverbs and prepositions also indicate position and direction. For example, position is indicated by *in* and *at*, and direction is indicated by *to* and *upwards*.
    Write out the following sentences and choose suitable verbs from Table 1 to to complete them. Usually more than one verb may be suitable. The prepositions and adverbs in the sentences indicate whether a verb of location or a verb of direction is required.

1. The heart ... above the diaphragm.
2. The lungs ... on either side of the heart.
3. The trachea ... from the pharynx to the junction of the main bronchi.
4. The oesophagus ... downwards.
5. The oesophagus ... downwards to the stomach.
6. The oesophagus ... downwards from the pharynx to the stomach.
7. The trachea ... anterior to the oesophagus.
8. The liver ... below the diaphragm.
9. The optic nerve ... from the retina into the cranial cavity.
10. The biconvex lens ... behind the iris.
11. The aorta ... through the diaphragm.
12. The Eustachian tube ... downwards from the middle ear and ... into the pharynx.

EXERCISE D *Locative prepositions*

Tables 2 and 3 below give some other verbs in common use, together with the prepositions which occur with them.

TABLE 2

reach meet join enter pierce	+Direct Object (i.e. no preposition)

TABLE 3

arise spring	+from, out of
originate	+from
give	+off
open	+into, on to, out of
start begin end	+at

NOTE. The prepositions above are the most usual with these verbs.
    Other prepositions may occur.

Write out the following sentences, and complete them with suitable prepositions. Sometimes no preposition is required. Tables 1, 2 and 3 should help you.

1. The heart lies ... the thoracic cavity.
2. The ulna extends ... the elbow ... the wrist.
3. The liver is ... the diaphragm.
4. The heart is situated ... the stomach.
5. The aorta gives ... the right and left coronary arteries.
6. The ileum is found ... the lower part of the abdomen.
7. The lingual nerve enters ... the mouth from outside the pharynx.
8. The urinary bladder is located ... the pelvis.
9. The ureters lead ... the kidneys ... the bladder.
10. The oesophagus descends ... the stomach.
11. The oesophagus descends to end ... the stomach.
12. The lungs lie ... the thorax.
13. The nostrils open ... the pharynx.
14. The lungs extend ... about one inch above the collarbone ... the diaphragm.
15. The kidneys are found ... the posterior part of the abdomen.
16. The spleen lies ... the stomach and the duodenum.
17. The vermiform appendix springs ... the caecum.

18. The bile duct joins ... the pancreatic duct and together they open ... the duodenum.
19. The femoral artery runs ... the inside of the thigh.
20. The dorsalis pedis gives ... branches to supply the dorsal side of the foot and toes.
21. The aorta pierces ... the diaphragm.
22. The jejunum is located ... the centre of the abdomen.
23. The ilio-psoas arises ... the lumbar vertebrae and the ilium.
24. The caecum starts ... the ileocaecal valve.
25. The small intestine meets ... the large intestine ... the ileocaecal valve.

EXERCISE E *Locative prefixes*

The following are some common locative prefixes.
    extra- (outside)   sub-   (below)
    intra- (inside)   infra- (below)
    inter- (between)   supra- (above)
    para- (beside)   retro- (behind)
    peri- (around)

Write out the following sentences, filling in the blanks in the right hand column.

(a) 1. fluid outside the cells   .... cellular fluid
     2. matrix between the cells   .... matrix
     3. pressure within the abdomen   .... -abdominal pressure
     4. gutter beside the colon   .... colic gutter
     5. compartment below the colon   infra ....
     6. membrane around the tooth   .... odontal ....
     7. duct between lobules   .... lobular duct
     8. vein within the liver   .... hepatic ....
     9. fossa beside the duodenum   .... duodenal ....
    10. fossa behind the duodenum   ....
    11. margin below the ribs   infracostal ....
    12. margin below the ribs   sub............................
    13. muscles between the ribs   ....
    14. nerve above the orbit   .... -orbital nerve
    15. nerve below the orbit   infra-...........................
    16. disc between the vertebrae   .... vertebral disc
    17. gutters beside the vertebrae   ....
    18. sinuses beside the nose   .... nasal ....
    19. fossa behind the caecum   .... caecal ....
    20. life within the uterus   .... -uterine ....
    21. region around the stomach   .... gastric ....
    22. arteries between bones   .... osseous ....

(b) 1. subcostal   below the ribs
2. intracellular ....
3. intermuscular ....
4. intermetacarpal ....
5. retroperitoneal ....
6. subepidermal ....
7. intravenous ....
8. pericaecal ....

III INFORMATION TRANSFER

1. Look at the following diagram and complete the exercises below it.

The stomach

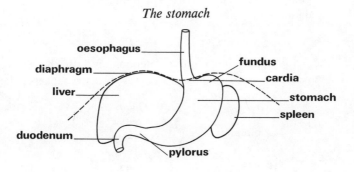

(a) Write out the following sentences, choosing the correct adjective from the pair in brackets at the end of each sentence.
1. The spleen lies ... to the stomach. (lateral, medial)
2. The liver is situated .... to the stomach. (superior, inferior)
3. The liver is situated ... to the diaphragm. (superior, inferior)
4. The pylorus is the ... opening of the stomach. (distal, lateral)
5. The fundus lies ... to the cardia. (anterior, superior)
6. The duodenum is the ... portion of the small intestine. (distal, proximal)

(b) Write out the following sentences, filling in the blanks with suitable prepositions.
The stomach lies ... the upper part of the abdominal cavity. It is inferior ... the diaphragm and liver and medial ... the spleen.
The stomach begins ... the cardia and extends downwards and to the right ... the pylorus.

2. Refer to the illustration and the notes below and write a brief account of the position of the oesophagus.

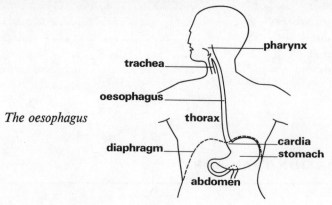

The oesophagus

Oesophagus long muscular tube – thorax – abdomen
trachea
pharynx – thoracic cavity – diaphragm
diaphragm – stomach – cardia

(4 sentences)

3. Write the paragraphs below in your notebook, and use the illustration to fill in the blanks. Sometimes a choice of words is given in brackets to help you.

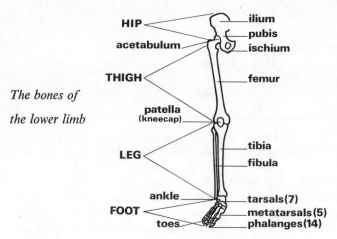

The bones of

the lower limb

The lower limb . . . . . . four main parts: the hip, ...
The hip bone is made up of three . . . . . . :   . . . .
The thigh bone, or . . . . . ., extends . . . . . . the hip . . . . the knee. Its . . . . . (upper, distal) end fits into the acetabulum.
The patella, ... kneecap, is a small bone which protects the knee joint. The knee joint . . . . the lower end of the . . . ., the kneecap, and the upper . . . . . . of the . . . . . .

The leg proper . . . . . . from the . . . . . . the ankle. It . . . . . . two bones:
namely the . . . . . . and the . . . . . . The tibia lies on the . . . . . . (medial,
lateral) side of the leg. The fibula . . . . . . on the . . . . . . of the leg. The fibula
takes no part in the formation of the knee joint. The . . . . . . (distal, proximal)
ends of both the tibia and the fibula form the . . . . (upper, lower) and
outer bones of the ankle.

The foot can be divided into . . . . parts. 7 tarsal bones . . . . . . the ankle
region. The middle part of the foot . . . . 5 metatarsal bones, and 14 . . . . . .
the bones of the . . . .

IV GUIDED WRITING

STAGE 1 *Sentence building*

Join each of the groups of sentences below into one longer sentence, using the
additional words printed in capital letters above some of the groups. Omit
words in italics. In addition, you may use relative clauses, short-form relative
clauses and *and*, omitting words when necessary.

1. The pericardium is conical in shape.
   It is fused at its apex with the roots of the great veins and arteries.
   It is fused at its base with the central tendon of the diaphragm.

2. TO COVER
   A layer of serous membrane lines the fibrous pericardium.
   It is reflected round the roots of the great veins and arteries.
   It covers the surface of the heart.

3. The pericardium is a fibrous sac.
   This fibrous sac encloses the heart.

4. The heart is separated from the fibrous pericardial sac.
   They are separated by two adjacent layers of serous membrane.

5. The pericardium is attached to the upper and lower ends of the sternum.
   It is attached by ligaments.

6. The pleura lines the thoracic wall.
   It also lines the upper surface of the diaphragm.
   It also lines the mediastinal surface.

7. The lungs and the pleural cavities are lined by the pleura.
   The pleura is a membrane of fibrous tissue.
   It is surfaced by a single layer of squamous epithelium.

8. JUST AS/AND AGAIN
   Each lung lies enclosed in a pleural sac.
   The heart lies *similarly* enclosed in the pericardial sac.
   Two layers of serous membrane are adjacent.

9. TO FORM
   At each lung root the pleura is reflected from the mediastinum.
   It forms a layer.
   The layer covers the surface of the lung.

STAGE 2 *Paragraph building*

Add the following material to the sentences indicated:

write 'thus' at the beginning of sentence 4
in sentence 5 change 'the pericardium' to 'it'
write 'in each cavity' at the beginning of sentence 6
write 'thus' at the beginning of sentence 8.

The sentences can be rearranged to make two paragraphs. Arrange sentences
1–5 in a logical order to form a paragraph about the pericardium. Arrange
sentences 6–9 in a logical order to make a similar paragraph about the pleura.

Compare your paragraphs with the relevant paragraphs in the Free Reading
section. Make any changes that you think are necessary, but remember that
sentences can often be arranged in more than one way.

STAGE 3 *Paragraph reconstruction*

Read through your paragraphs again. Make sure you know all the words,
using a dictionary if necessary. Without referring to your previous work,
rewrite the paragraphs. Here are some notes to help you.

paragraph 1
   pericardium – fibrous sac – encloses heart
   conical shape – fused at apex – roots of great veins and arteries – fused at
      base – central tendon of diaphragm
   attached by ligaments – upper and lower ends of sternum
   layer of serous membrane – fibrous pericardium – reflected round roots of
      great veins and arteries – covers surface of heart
   heart separated from fibrous pericardial sac – two adjacent layers of serous
      membrane

paragraph 2
   lungs and pleural cavities – pleura – membrane of fibrous tissue – single
      layer of squamous epithelium
   in each cavity – pleura – thoracic wall – upper surface of diaphragm –
      mediastinal surface

at each lung root – pleura reflected from mediastinum – covers surface of
   lung
each lung enclosed in pleural sac – heart in pericardial sac – two layers of
   serous membrane adjacent

V FREE READING

Read the following passage in your own time. Try to find additional examples
of the points you have studied in this and other units.

The Thoracic Cavity

The *thoracic cavity* is divided by fibrous partitions into three compartments.
The central compartment, the *mediastinum*, is a mass of tissue and organs,
extending from the vertebral column behind to the sternum in front. It contains the heart and great blood vessels, the oesophagus, the trachea and its
bifurcation, the phrenic and vagus nerves, and the thoracic duct. The two
lateral compartments are cavities, known as the *pleural cavities*. These contain the lungs.

The *mediastinum* is commonly considered to have three divisions, lying
anterior, posterior and superior to the *pericardium*. Both the anterior and
the posterior mediastinum are continuous with the superior mediastinum,
which connects freely with the neck.

The *anterior mediastinum* is not much more than a potential space. It lies
between the sternum and the pericardium and is overlapped by the anterior
edges of both lungs. It sometimes contains the lower part of the thymus
gland, but usually this does not extend lower than the superior mediastinum.

The *posterior mediastinum* lies behind the pericardium and the diaphragm.
It contains the thoracic lymph nodes and, in addition, various organs in
their passage to or from the superior mediastinum. These are principally the
aorta and the oesophagus, which descend from the superior mediastinum
through the posterior mediastinum to the abdomen, and the thoracic duct,
which leads upwards from the posterior mediastinum into the superior
mediastinum.

The *superior mediastinum* contains the oesophagus, the trachea, the
apices of the lungs, the phrenic and vagus nerves, the arch of the aorta, and
other major blood vessels. The superior mediastinum is remarkable for the
asymetrical relationships of its contents, mainly due to the position of the
great veins and arteries, i.e. veins on the right side and arteries on the left.
The trachea, for example, is in contact with the right vagus nerve and the
apex of the right lung, but is separated from the left vagus and the apex of
the left lung by the left common carotid and the left subclavian arteries.

The *pericardium* is a fibrous sac which encloses the heart. The pericardium is conical in shape, fused at its apex with the roots of the great veins and arteries and at its base with the central tendon of the diaphragm. It is attached by ligaments to the upper and lower ends of the sternum. A layer of serous membrane lines the fibrous pericardium and is reflected round the roots of the great veins and arteries to cover the surface of the heart. Thus the heart is separated from the fibrous pericardial sac by two adjacent layers of serous membrane.

The lungs and the *pleural cavities* are lined by the pleura, a membrane of fibrous tissue surfaced by a single layer of squamous epithelium. In each cavity the pleura lines the thoracic wall, the upper surface of the diaphragm and the mediastinal surface. At each lung root the pleura is reflected from the mediastinum to form a layer which covers the surface of the lung. Thus each lung lies enclosed in a pleural sac, just as the heart lies enclosed in the pericardial sac, and again two layers of serous membrane are adjacent.

The pericardium and the pleura have the same function, namely to provide two slippery surfaces so that the structures contained within can move without friction. The thoracic cavity is a very mobile area. The heart is in rhythmic pulsation and changes its position a little between systole and diastole; the lungs also are in rhythmic motion, gliding down and up; the oesophagus dilates with each bolus; and the great veins expand considerably during increased blood flow.

4 Epithelial Tissue

I READING AND COMPREHENSION

[1]Epithelial tissue lines the body internally and covers it externally. [2]It is generally attached to a basement membrane of fibrous tissue. [3]Internally it lines both mucous and serous membranes. [4]Externally it overlies the dermis to form the outer layer of the skin, or epidermis.

[5]The cells of epithelial tissue are situated continuously. [6]There is virtually no intercellular matrix. [7]The cells may form one or more layers. [8]When the cells lie in a single layer the epithelium is said to be simple. [9]When the cells form several layers the epithelium is said to be stratified.

(a) Epithelial tissue is a basement membrane.
(b) Mucous membrane is composed of epithelial tissue.
(c) The epidermis is composed of epithelial tissue.
(d) The cells of epithelial tissue are scattered through an intercellular matrix.
(e) Simple epithelium has one or more layers of cells.

[10]There are various types of simple epithelium, classified mainly according to cell shape. [11]*Pavement epithelium* is a simple epithelium with flattened cells lying edge to edge. [12]It makes the smooth surface lining the serous membranes of the pleura, pericardium and peritoneum. [13]It is found also wherever a very thin membrane is required, e.g. in the terminal vesicles of the renal tubules. [14]*Columnar epithelium* is a simple epithelium composed of column-shaped cells. [15]These are again arranged edge to edge. [16]Columnar epithelium lines the mucous membrane of the stomach and the intestines. [17]It also lines the gall-bladder and bile ducts, and the ducts of several glands. [18]The height of the columnar cells varies from region to region. [19]In some parts of the body, such as inside the convoluted portion of the renal tubules, the cells are so low that their height equals their width. [20]The epithelium is then called *cubical epithelium*. [21]In other regions a protoplasmic 'hair' may be attached to each columnar cell. [22]These hairs are known as 'cilia' and the epithelium is referred to as *columnar ciliated epithelium*. [23]Columnar ciliated epithelium is found in many parts of the body, but most notably in the nasal cavities.

(f) Pavement epithelium has only one layer.

(g) Cubical epithelium is found inside the convoluted portion of the renal tubules.

(h) Columnar ciliated epithelium is found only in the nasal cavities.

[24]The most important stratified epithelium is *stratified squamous epithelium*, which forms the epidermis. [25]As its cells approach the surface they gradually lose their protoplasmic contents and become flatter and more scale-like (squamous). [26]At the same time the cells in the superficial layers are gradually converted into keratin, especially in the palmar and plantar regions. [27]Stratified squamous epithelium also lines the oral cavity, the lower part of the pharynx, the oesophagus, the anal canal and the vagina. [28]In these areas there is little keratin and the epithelium is not so thick.

[29]Other types of stratified epithelium are found: for example, layers of conical and oval cells lie deep to a layer of columnar ciliated cells in the epithelium lining the mucous membrane of the trachea and the bronchi.

(i) There are various types of stratified epithelium.

(j) The epithelium in the palmar and plantar regions contains little keratin.

(k) The epithelium in the oesophagus contains little keratin.

(l) Stratified squamous epithelium lines the mucous membrane of the trachea and the bronchi.

Solutions

(a) It (epithelial tissue) is generally ATTACHED TO a basement membrane. (2)

i.e. epithelial tissue $\neq$ a basement membrane.

∴ It is NOT TRUE that epithelial tissue is a basement membrane.

(b) Internally it (epithelial tissue) lines both mucous and serous membranes. (3)

i.e. Mucous membrane is covered with a layer of epithelial tissue.

∴ It is NOT TRUE that mucous membrane is composed of epithelial tissue.

(c) Externally it (epithelial tissue) overlies the dermis to form the outer layer of the skin, or epidermis. (4)

i.e. Epithelial tissue forms the outer layer of the skin, or epidermis
= Epithelial tissue forms the epidermis.

∴ *The epidermis is composed of epithelial tissue.*

(d) The cells of epithelial tissue are situated continuously. (5)

i.e. The cells of epithelial tissue are NOT scattered.
There is virtually no intercellular matrix. (6)

∴ It is NOT TRUE that the cells of epithelial tissue are scattered through an intercellular matrix.

(e) When the cells lie in a single layer the epithelium is said to be simple. (8)

i.e. Simple epithelium has only a single layer of cells.

∴ It is NOT TRUE that simple epithelium has one or more layers of cells.

(f) Pavement epithelium is a simple epithelium. (11)

Simple epithelium has only one layer. (see 8)

∴ *Pavement epithelium has only one layer.*

(g) The epithelium is then called cubical epithelium. (20)

then = when the cells are so low that their height equals their width (see 19)

i.e. Cubical epithelium occurs in some parts of the body, such as inside the convoluted portion of the renal tubules. (see 19)

∴ *Cubical epithelium is found inside the convoluted portion of the renal tubules.*

(h) Columnar ciliated epithelium is found in many parts of the body. (23)

∴ It is NOT TRUE that columnar ciliated epithelium is found ONLY in the nasal cavities.

(i) The most important stratified epithelium is stratified squamous epithelium. (24)

Other types of stratified epithelium are found. (29)

∴ *There are various types of stratified epithelium.*

(j) The cells in the superficial layers are gradually converted into keratin, especially in the palmar and plantar regions. (26)

i.e. The superficial layers of stratified squamous epithelium contain keratin, especially in the palmar and plantar regions.

i.e. The epithelium in the palmar and plantar regions contains most keratin.

∴ It is NOT TRUE that the epithelium in the palmar and plantar regions contains little keratin.

(k) In these areas there is little keratin. (28)

these areas = the oral cavity, the lower part of the pharynx, the oesophagus, the anal canal and the vagina (27)

∴ *The epithelium in the oesophagus contains little keratin.*

(l)   Other types of stratified epithelium are found: for example, ... the epithelium lining the mucous membrane of the trachea and the bronchi. (29)

other = not squamous (see 24)

∴   It is NOT TRUE that stratified squamous epithelium lines the mucous membrane of the trachea and the bronchi.

EXERCISE A *Contextual reference*

What do the following refer to?

1. 'it' in sentence 3
2. 'it' in sentence 12
3. 'these' in sentence 15
4. 'it' in sentence 17
5. 'their' in sentence 19
6. 'these areas' in sentence 28

EXERCISE B *Rephrasing*

Rewrite the following sentences, replacing the words printed in italics with expressions from the reading passage which have the same meaning.

1. *Epithelium* is *usually* attached to fibrous tissue.
2. The epidermis *lies superior to* the dermis.
3. In pavement epithelium the cells *lie edge to edge*.
4. There is *little or no* intercellular matrix in epithelial tissue.
5. The cells may *form* several layers.
6. There are various *kinds* of epithelium.
7. Cubical epithelium is *made up of* cubical cells.
8. Pavement epithelium is sometimes *known* as tesselated epithelium.
9. In some *regions* the epithelium is ciliated.
10. The height of the cells *is different in different regions*.
11. The cells on the surface are *squamous*.
12. The cells are gradually *keratinized*.
13. The keratin is quite thick, *particularly* in areas of great wear and tear.
14. Layers of cells lie *below* a layer of ciliated cells.

EXERCISE C *Relationships between statements*

Place one of the expressions below in each of the sentences indicated. Where necessary, replace and re-order the words in the sentences, and change the punctuation.

consequently   in addition   however

(6) (17) (28) (22) (13)

II USE OF LANGUAGE

EXERCISE A *Verbs of naming*

(a) Copy the following table into your notebook and refer to the reading passage to complete it.

EPITHELIUM

Type	*Name*
1. several layers of cells 2. several layers of cells, the superficial layer being squamous 3. a single layer of flattened cells 4. a single layer of columnar cells 5. a single layer of columnar cells with 'hairs' attached 6. a single layer of cubical cells	stratified epithelium

(b) Refer to the completed table and write sentences naming the types of epithelium. Begin each sentence: *Epithelium which consists of* ... Use any of the following verbs:

is named is known as
is called is referred to as

EXAMPLE

Epithelium which consists of several layers of cells is named stratified epithelium.

(c) Verbs of naming are frequently found in past participle form, in a short-form relative clause.

EXAMPLE

Sound waves are conveyed through a curved canal known as the external auditory meatus.

Another way of naming is simply to add the name, separated from the rest of the sentence by comas.

EXAMPLE

Sound waves are conveyed through a curved canal, the external auditory meatus.

Name the structures shown in italics in the following sentences. The names are given in brackets. Use a short-form relative clause with any of the verbs of naming given in section (b) above; or simply add the name, separated from the rest of the sentence by commas.

EXAMPLE
　　　The eyeball lies in *a socket* (the orbit).
=　The eyeball lies in a socket called the orbit.
OR　The eyeball lies in a socket, the orbit.

1. Within the vestibule of the ear there are *two membranous sacs* (the utricle and the saccule).
2. *Large, pale phagocytic cells* (histiocytes) are found in the medulla of a lymph node.
3. The canal of the spinal cord widens out when it reaches the brain to form *a system of cavities* (the ventricles).
4. The peripheral edge of the acetabulum is deepened by *a rim* (the labrum acetabulare).
5. Scattered between the lobules of the pancreas are *clumps of cells* (the islets of Langerhans).
6. The alveoli of the lungs are lined by a *type of epithelium* (pavement epithelium).
7. The small bile ducts within the liver join up to form *one duct* (the hepatic duct).
8. A shallow socket at the proximal end of the radius moves round *a fixed ball* (the capitulum).
9. The pleura surrounding the lung root hangs down in *an empty fold* (the pulmonary ligament).
10. The medulla of the thymic lobule is made up of *small round cells* (thymocytes).

EXERCISE B *Naming by* or

Another way of naming a structure is to add *or* + name, separated from the rest of the sentence by commas. Notice that when *or* is used, the definite article is usually omitted.

EXAMPLE
　These folds of membrane, or vocal cords, stretch across the cavity of the larynx from front to back.

Using *or*, name the structures shown in italics in the following sentences. Do not use the definite article in front of the name.

EXAMPLE
   Epithelium forms *the superficial layer of the skin* (the epidermis).
= Epithelium forms the superficial layer of the skin, or epidermis.

1. *Cartilage-destroying cells* (osteoclasts) invade the cartilage and eat away the matrix.
2. The ileum has in its wall opposite the mesentery *distinctive patches of lymphoid tissue* (Peyer's patches).
3. Between the central nervous system and the surrounding bone there are *three membranes* (the meninges).
4. The notochord expands to form *the gelatinous centre of the intervertebral disc* (the nucleus pulposus).
5. *A thick layer of bony substance* (dentine) lies within the enamel of the tooth.
6. An artery has *an outer fibrous coat* (the tunica adventitia), *a middle muscular coat* (the tunica media), and *an inner endothelial coat* (the tunica interna).

EXERCISE C *The present participle and the past participle as modifiers*
The present participle (the *-ing* form of the verb) and the past participle (the *-ed* form of the verb) can be used like adjectives to modify a noun.

EXAMPLES
   the *developing* embryo
= the embryo which is developing
   a *distended* bladder
= a bladder which is distended
   newly formed lymphocytes
= lymphocytes which have been newly formed.

NOTE
 (i) the *-ing* form is derived from an active verb.
 (ii) the *-ed* form is derived from a passive verb.
 (iii) The choice between the *-ing* and the *-ed* form depends on active/passive, NOT on tense.
 (iv) The adverb must go before the verb form.

Convert the following relative clauses to participle modifiers:
 1. a thyroid gland which is enlarged
 2. a gland which secretes
 3. heat loss which has been reduced
 4. a diet which is properly balanced
 5. membranous tissue which intervenes
 6. muscles which contract
 7. cells which are scattered widely
 8. a blood sugar concentration which is rising
 9. the ends which have been expanded
 10. a valve which is functioning

EXERCISE D *Participles as modifiers and short-form relative clauses*
Join each of the following pairs of sentences into one sentence. Whenever
possible, change the verb in the second sentence into a participle modifying
a noun in the first sentence.

EXAMPLE
    The juices help the process of digestion. The juices are secreted.
=   The secreted juices help the process of digestion.

When this is not possible, change the second sentence into a short-form relative clause after a noun in the first sentence.

EXAMPLE
    The juices help the process of digestion. The juices are secreted by the
    stomach.
=   The juices secreted by the stomach help the process of digestion.

1. Glucose is taken out of the bloodstream by the muscles. The glucose has
   been reabsorbed.
2. There is a piece of cartilage between an epiphysis and a bone shaft. The
   cartilage grows.
3. A pulmonary artery enters each lung. A pulmonary artery contains de-
   oxygenated blood.
4. The intestine receives food. The food is partly digested.
5. The pericardium is a sac. This sac surrounds the heart.
6. The soft gland is known as the pancreas. The soft gland extends from the
   liver to the spleen.
7. Elastic tissue contains fibres. The fibres branch.
8. The periosteum is a membrane of fibrous tissue. This membrane of fibrous
   tissue tightly clothes the bone.
9. Slight lack of oxygen in the air has little effect on man. The air is inspired.
10. The diaphragm is a dome-shaped muscle. This dome-shaped muscle sepa-
    rates the thorax from the abdomen.
11. The surfaces are covered by hyaline cartilage. The surfaces articulate.
12. The medulla has 12–16 conical processes. These processes project into the
    pelvis.

EXERCISE E *Anatomical terms* (surround, line, surface, *etc.*)
Write out the following sentences, choosing the most suitable word to complete each sentence.

1. The pavement epithelium lies on a basement ...
   (a) layer
   (b) surface
   (c) membrane

2. The endocardium is a serous membrane which ... the heart cavities.
   (a) coats
   (b) lines
   (c) surrounds

3. Arterial walls have three ...
   (a) coats
   (b) surfaces
   (c) linings

4. The fat cells form a lobule, which is ... by a fibrous sheath.
   (a) lined
   (b) enclosed
   (c) attached

5. Areolar tissue contains a ... of branching fibres.
   (a) network
   (b) lining
   (c) sac

6. The epidermis is ... the dermis by a basement membrane.
   (a) attached to
   (b) lined by
   (c) invested in

7. Small cavities, called lacunae, ... the bone cells.
   (a) overlie
   (b) contain
   (c) surround

8. The ... of the epidermis consists of keratinized squamous cells.
   (a) surface
   (b) layer
   (c) lining

9. In the medulla oblongata, the nerve cells are ... to form a fluted rod.
   (a) lined
   (b) attached
   (c) arranged

10. A single ... of cells lines the intestinal mucous membrane.
    (a) surface
    (b) layer
    (c) lining

11. The crown of a tooth is ... with enamel.
    (a) coated
    (b) lined
    (c) enclosed

12. The entoderm forms the ... of the alimentary cavity.
   (a) network
   (b) lining
   (c) layer

13. A serous membrane ... cavities which do not communicate with the outside of the body.
   (a) covers
   (b) surrounds
   (c) lines

14. Concentric layers of bony matrix ... a central canal.
   (a) line
   (b) surround
   (c) contain

15. Sarcoplasm is surrounded by a ... of sarcolemma.
   (a) surface
   (b) wall
   (c) cavity

III   INFORMATION TRANSFER

1. Refer to the diagram and write out the paragraph, using the verbs given below. Use each verb once, and keep in mind that the verbs may be active or passive.

Section of a movable joint

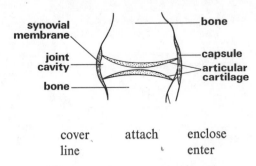

cover   attach   enclose
line   enter

   The joint cavity ...... by the capsule, which consists of strong fibrous tissue. Articular cartilage, to which the capsule ......, ... the surface of the bone which ...... the cavity. The inside of the cavity ...... by synovial membrane, which secretes a viscous fluid.

2. Refer to the diagram and write out the following paragraph.

Section of the brain and meninges

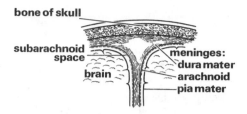

bone of skull

subarachnoid
space

brain

meninges:
dura mater
arachnoid
pia mater

Three membranes ...... the meninges lie between the ...... and the bone of the skull. The meninges ...... the pia mater, ... The pia mater is a vascular membrane ...... the brain very closely. The dura mater lines the ...... and gives ...... septa, which partly divide the cranial cavity. The arachnoid ...... between ...... It is a serous ...... which secretes the cerebrospinal fluid filling the cranial ......

3. Describe the structure of the integument of a leg, referring to the diagram and completing the paragraph below it. Write the paragraph in your note-book.

Section through the integument of a leg

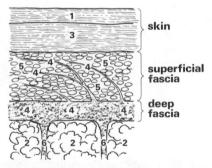

skin

superficial
fascia

deep
fascia

1. epidermis 2. muscles 3. corium, or dermis
4. collagenous tissue 5. fatty tissue
6. intermuscular septa

This section through the ...... of a leg shows the different fascial layers. Above is the skin, consisting of the .... to the skin lies the ......, which is made up of ...... supported by delicate layers of ...... The deep fascia, ... below the ......, consists of a dense layer of ...... From the .... processes extend downwards among the ...... to form ......

IV GUIDED WRITING

STAGE 1 *Sentence building*

Join each of the groups of sentences below into one longer sentence, using the additional words printed in capital letters above some of the groups. Omit words in italics. You may also use relative clauses, short-form relative clauses, *and* and *but*, and you may omit words where necessary.

1. Fat cells are normally arranged to form a lobule.
   The lobule is enclosed by a delicate collagenous sheath.

2. REMOVING
   Histiocytes have the power of amoeboid movement.
   Histiocytes may move about the tissue.
   Histiocytes remove cell debris from the tissue spaces.

3. Fat cells consist mainly of a large droplet of fat.
   The large droplet of fat is surrounded by a thin envelope of cytoplasm.

4. WITH
   Fibroblasts are flat cells.
   Fibroblasts are star-shaped cells.
   Fibroblasts have a large nucleus and fairly clear cytoplasm.

5. I.E./THEY
   Histiocytes have phagocytic properties.
   Histiocytes are able to ingest foreign material.

6. Various types of cell are found in connective tissue.
   The most important of these cells are the fibroblasts, histiocytes and fat cells.

7. SO/THAT
   The cells are usually swollen with the fat.
   The nucleus is pushed to one side.

8. Fibroblasts are stationary cells.
   Fibroblasts are concerned with the production of collagenous fibres.

9. Histiocytes have a smaller nucleus than that of the fibroblasts.
   The cytoplasm is generally filled with granules and vacuoles.
   The vacuoles are a result of their phagocytic activity.

STAGE 2 *Paragraph building*

Rewrite the nine sentences in a logical order, to make a paragraph, making the following changes to the sentences indicated:

write 'they' instead of 'histiocytes' in sentence 2
add 'also' to sentence 2
add 'on the other hand' to sentence 5
write 'they' instead of 'fibroblasts' in sentence 8.

When you have written your paragraph, re-read it and make sure the sentences are presented in a logical order. Give the paragraph you have written a suitable title. Compare your paragraph with the relevant paragraph in the Free Reading section. Make any changes that you think are necessary, but remember that sentences can often be arranged in more than one way.

STAGE 3 *Paragraph reconstruction*

Read through your paragraph again. Make sure you know all the words, using a dictionary if necessary. Without referring to your previous work, re-write the paragraph. Here are some notes to help you.

various types of cell in connective tissue
fibroblasts
flat, star-shaped – large nucleus – fairly clear cytoplasm
stationary – concerned with production of collagenous fibres
histiocytes
phagocytic properties – can ingest foreign material
amoeboid movement – move about tissue – remove cell debris – tissue
  spaces
smaller nucleus – cytoplasm filled with granules – vacuoles – result of
  phagocytic activity
fat cells
mainly large droplet of fat – thin envelope of cytoplasm
swollen – nucleus pushed to one side
normally arranged in lobule – delicate collagenous sheath

V FREE READING

Read the following passage in your own time. Try to find additional examples of the points you have studied in this and other units.

Connective Tissue

Connective tissue is primarily the supporting tissue of the body, acting as a packing material and binding together the various bodily structures. There are several types of connective tissue, but all are characterized by a large amount of intercellular matrix, which is mainly of a fibrous nature. The cells which are scattered throughout the tissue are important only in that they produce and maintain the matrix, and it is according to the structure and consistency of the matrix that the tissues are classified.

The fibres found in connective tissue are chiefly of two kinds, collagenous and elastic. Collagenous fibres are delicate wavy fibres which individually present an almost colourless appearance but in mass make up a white tissue. The tissue is very tough, and particularly resistant to tensile stress. The fibres are arranged in bundles, within which they run a wavy course parallel to each other. Elastic fibres are yellow in colour, and unlike the white fibres they run singly, branching frequently and anastomosing with each other.

Various types of cell are found in connective tissue, but the most important of these are the fibroblasts, histiocytes and fat cells. Fibroblasts are flat, star-shaped cells with a large nucleus and fairly clear cytoplasm. They are stationary cells, concerned with the production of collagenous fibres. Histiocytes, on the other hand, have phagocytic properties, i.e. they are able to ingest foreign material. They have also the power of amoeboid movement, and may move about the tissue, removing cell debris from the tissue spaces. Histiocytes have a smaller nucleus than that of the fibroblasts, and the cytoplasm is generally filled with granules and vacuoles, which are a result of their phagocytic activity. Fat cells consist mainly of a large droplet of fat, surrounded by a thin envelope of cytoplasm. The cells are usually so swollen with the fat that the nucleus is pushed to one side. Fat cells are normally arranged to form a lobule, which is enclosed by a delicate collagenous sheath.

Fat cells are found in a tissue of few fibres, called adipose tissue. This is found in specific areas of the body, e.g. the superficial fascia and the mesenteries of the peritoneum.

Other kinds of connective tissue are largely differentiated by the amount and proportion of the collagenous and elastic fibres they contain. Collagenous fibres are found pure in tendons and elastic fibres are found almost pure in certain ligaments, but most connective tissue is made up of a mixture of collagenous and elastic fibres, with collagenous fibres predominating. The total amount of fibres varies also. A loose network of white and yellow fibres lying on a gelatinous base is known as areolar tissue. Areolar tissue lies between structures, holding them in place. Sheaths, septa and capsules surrounding various muscles, glands, etc. are formed by a very dense fibrous tissue.

Cartilage and bone are commonly considered to be very firm connective tissue. The fibres in cartilage lie in a ground substance which is rubbery and resilient. The matrix of bone is hardened by lime salts, mainly calcium phosphate.

5 The Study of Cell Structure

---

[1]The general structure of tissues and organs has been studied for a long time. [2]It is now fairly well understood. [3]This is not the case with the study of cell structure, which is comparatively new. [4]Cytology is particularly dependent on the development of new examination techniques. [5]These techniques are largely sophisticated methods of light microscopy, but recently the electron microscope has been added to the tools of research.

[6]All methods of microscopy have two functions. [7]They must give a magnified image with a high degree of resolution, or definition of detail. [8]In addition, they must achieve a sharp contrast between the specimen and its environment, so that the specimen is clearly visible. [9]Light microscopy functions by exploitation of the properties of light waves. [10]The image is formed because of the ability of an object to absorb, reflect or refract light waves. [11]The electron microscope uses a beam of electrons instead of light waves.

(a) Cell structure is now fairly well understood.
(b) The functions of microscopy are magnification, resolution and contrast.
(c) To resolve an image is to show its individual parts clearly.
(d) Light microscopy functions by the absorption, reflection and refraction of light waves.

[12]It is customary to divide the development of cytology into three periods. [13]From 1875 to 1900, the nucleus of the cell and the process of mitosis were studied, often by using an achromatic lens. [14]This is a lens which refracts white light without breaking it up into its component colours. [15]The apochromatic lens in use nowadays is still more highly corrected for colour aberrations.

[16]In the period from 1900 to 1940 more precise methods of fixing and staining became available to researchers and methods of light microscopy were improved. [17]A fresh awareness of Mendel's work led to the study of chromosomes and genetics from 1900 to 1925. [18]From 1925 to 1940 interest centred on the cytoplasm. [19]It had already been ascertained that the cell

consists of a nucleus, contained by a nuclear membrane, and cytoplasm, which occupies the rest of the cell. [20]By 1940 certain features of the cytoplasm were detectable, including the cylindrical centrioles, but much was postulated and investigations were limited by the techniques available.

(e) The achromatic lens, like the apochromatic, is used to correct colour aberrations.

(f) Mendel studied chromosomes and genetics from 1900 to 1925.

(g) The cell consists of two major parts.

[21]A new era of cytology began in 1940. [22]The development of the ultra-microtome for cutting extremely thin sections made the electron microscope applicable to cell study. [23]The cytoplasmic matrix appeared homogeneous with the phase contrast technique of light microscopy. [24]However, the EM, or electron microscope, showed that it is divided by membranes into compartments with different chemical constitutions. [25]The EM was essential to the investigation of the endoplasmic reticulum and the ribosomes. [26]It also revealed in fine detail the mitochondria, the cilia, the Golgi complex and the cylindrical centrioles.

(h) The EM was not invented until 1940.

(i) The cytoplasmic matrix is homogeneous.

(j) The cylindrical centrioles were first detected by the EM.

[27]All techniques have their own limitations. [28]Cells growing in culture may be different from cells in intact tissue. [29]Because of technical difficulties of staining, the EM has shown very little about nuclear structure. [30]The information provided by all the available techniques of structural examination must be combined, and experimental techniques using ultraviolet light, fluorescence and sensitive television cameras must be perfected. [31]Thus our understanding of cell structure will be increased.

(k) The EM is limited in its study of nuclear structure.

(l) Our understanding of cell structure will be increased only by perfecting experimental techniques.

Solutions

(a) It is now fairly well understood. (2)
    it = the general structure of tissues and organs
    This is not the case with the study of cell structure. (3)
∴   It is NOT TRUE that cell structure is fairly well understood.

(b) All methods of microscopy have two functions. (6)
    (i) They must give a magnified image with a high degree of resolution. (7)

(ii) They must achieve a sharp contrast. (8)

i.e. *The functions of microscopy are magnification, resolution and contrast.*

(c) They must give a magnified image with a high degree of resolution, or definition of detail. (7)

    resolution = definition of detail

    to define detail = to show individual parts clearly

∴ *To resolve an image is to show its individual parts clearly.*

(d) Light microscopy functions by exploitation of the properties of light waves. (9)

    ... the ability of an object to absorb, reflect or refract light waves. (10)

i.e. *Light microscopy functions by the absorption, reflection and refraction of light waves.*

(e) The apochromatic lens ... is still more highly corrected for colour aberrations. (15)

    more highly = more highly than the achromatic lens (see 14)

i.e. The achromatic lens is highly corrected for colour aberrations, and the apochromatic lens is STILL MORE highly corrected.

∴ *The achromatic lens, like the apochromatic, is used to correct colour aberrations.*

(f) From 1900 to 1925 there was a fresh awareness of Mendel's work. (see 17)

    a fresh awareness = an awareness again

i.e. There had been an awareness of Mendel's work before 1900.

i.e. Mendel's work was done before 1900.

∴ It is NOT TRUE that Mendel studied chromosomes and genetics from 1900 to 1925. (Other researchers studied chromosomes and genetics during this period.)

(g) The cell consists of a nucleus, contained by the nuclear membrane, and cytoplasm, which occupies the rest of the cell. (19)

= The cell consists of

    (i) a nucleus, contained by the nuclear membrane

    (ii) cytoplasm, which occupies the rest of the cell.

i.e. *The cell consists of two major parts.*

(h) In 1940 the development of the ultramicrotome made the EM applicable to cell study. (see 21 and 22)

i.e. The EM was invented before 1940, but could not be used for cell study until 1940.

∴ It is NOT TRUE that the EM was not invented until 1940.

(i)   The cytoplasmic matrix appeared homogeneous. (23)
        appeared ≠ is
        The EM showed that it is divided into compartments with different
        chemical constitutions (see 24)
i.e.   The cytoplasmic matrix is NOT homogeneous.

(j)   By 1940 certain features of the cytoplasm were detectable, including the
        cylindrical centrioles. (20)
        It (the EM) revealed in fine detail the ... cylindrical centrioles. (26)
i.e.   The cylindrical centrioles were first detected by light microscopy before
        1940; after 1940 the EM revealed them in more detail.
∴   'The cylindrical centrioles were NOT first detected by the EM.

(k)   Because of technical difficulties of staining, the EM has shown VERY
        LITTLE about nuclear structure. (29)
∴   *The EM is limited in its study of nuclear structure.*

(l)   Thus our understanding of cell structure will be increased. (31)
        thus = (i) by combining the information provided by all the available
                      techniques (see 30)
              (ii) by perfecting experimental techniques (see 30)
∴   Our understanding of cell structure will NOT be increased ONLY by per-
        fecting experimental techniques.

EXERCISE A *Contextual reference*

Write the following sentences in your notebook and complete them after
studying the reading passage.
1. 'it' in sentence 2 refers to ......
2. 'which' in sentence 3 refers to ......
3. 'they' in sentence 8 refers to ......
4. 'this' in sentence 14 refers to ......
5. 'it' in sentence 24 refers to ......
6. 'it' in sentence 26 refers to ......

EXERCISE B *Rephrasing*

Rewrite the following sentences, replacing the words printed in italics with expressions from the reading passage which have the same meaning.
1. The development of new techniques is *especially* important in cytology.
2. *Highly developed* methods of light microscopy are *being used* now.
3. A phase contrast microscope, like all light microscopes, *works* by *making use of* light waves.
4. The achromatic lens helps to prevent *distortions of colour*.
5. The cytoplasmic matrix *presented a homogeneous appearance* in the phase
   contrast microscope.
6. The EM *revealed* the Golgi complex in fine detail.

7. Due to difficulties of staining, the *electron microscope* has contributed little to the *research* into nuclear structure.

EXERCISE C *Relationships between statements*

Put the following expressions in appropriate places in the paragraphs indicated. If necessary, replace and re-order the words in the sentences and change the punctuation.
(a) however (paragraph 1)
(b) firstly, secondly, i.e. (paragraph 2)
(c) in addition, then, nevertheless (paragraph 4)
(d) furthermore (paragraph 6)

II USE OF LANGUAGE

EXERCISE A study, use, improve, *etc.*

1. Copy the following table into your notebook and complete it with information from the reading passage.

THE DEVELOPMENT OF CYTOLOGY

Dates	Techniques available	Principal areas of study
1875–....	1. light microscopy 2. achromatic	1. .... 2. ....
....–....	improved methods of: 1. .... and .... 2.	1. .... and .... 2. ....
....–now	new tools: 1. .... 2.	1. .... matrix 2. .... and .... 3. details of ....
future	improved methods of: 1. .... 2. .... 3. .... perhaps also new techniques	nuclear structure?

2. Use the table and the words given below to complete the following sentences. Write the sentences in your notebook. The verbs are to be used in the passive. Choose a suitable tense.

   Nouns: study, use, development, improvement
   Verbs: study, use, develop, improve

(a) Mitosis ...... before 1900.
(b) Methods of fixing and staining ...... during the period ......
(c) The ...... of methods using ultraviolet light, ..., and ...... may advance the ...... of ......
(d) A detailed ...... of the cylindrical centrioles was not possible before ......
(e) The .... of cell structure .... considerably since 1875.
(f) Methods of ...... microscopy ...... in the .... of .... from .... to 1900.
(g) Now the ...... and the ...... are available for ...... in cell ......
(h) The ...... of new experimental techniques may advance the ......
(i) The electron microscope ...... to study the ....

EXERCISE B *Passives without an agent*

The passive voice of the verb can be used to describe a state rather than an action.

EXAMPLE
   The popliteal muscle is attached to the femur and tibia.

If the verb is made active, it is often difficult to imagine what the subject of the sentence would be, as in this example:

   X attaches the popliteal muscle to the femur and tibia.

This is because we are concerned with the state of attachment of the muscle, and not with the action of attaching it.

   Stative passives occur commonly in medical writing. They are always in the present tense. If you prefer, you can think of them as the verb *to be* + a past participle used adjectivally.

   Complete each of the following sentences by the stative passive of the verb in brackets at the end of the sentence.

1. The epidermis ... over the papillae of the dermis. (mould)
2. Osteoblasts ... from undifferentiated connective tissue cells. (derive)
3. Nerve fibres ... with a layer of myelin. (insulate)
4. The cavity of a tooth ... with pulp. (fill)
5. The patella ... in the tendon of the femur. (embed)
6. Molars ... for grinding food. (adapt)
7. Cellular elements ... in the blood. (isolate)
8. The sympathetic nerves ... throughout the body. (distribute)
9. The pectoralis minor ... into the coracoid process of the scapula. (insert)
10. The ribs ... in pairs. (arrange)

EXERCISE C *Passive with an agent, expressed or unexpressed*

Change the verbs in the following sentences from the active to the passive. When the agent is personal, omit it.

EXAMPLES
  (a) The nuclear membrane encloses DNA in the nucleus.
      DNA is enclosed in the nucleus by the nuclear membrane.
  (b) We divide lamellae into two types.
      Lamellae are divided into two types.

NOTE
  (i) Both the examples above are stative passives.
  (ii) Omission of the agent in example (b) serves to make the statement impersonal. Impersonality is another feature of medical writing.

1. Age, sex and function influence the rate of bone growth.
2. We call the eye socket the orbit.
3. When we add iodine solution to glycogen, we produce a port-wine colour.
4. Mucous membrane lines the intestinal tract.
5. The kidneys remove bilirubin from the blood.
6. Physiologists studied the process of mitosis at the end of the last century.
7. A delicate plexus of nerve fibres accompanies blood vessels.
8. Chemists extract quinine from cinchona.
9. We do not understand the function of the thymus.
10. The quadriceps muscle supports the front of the knee.
11. Lack of oxygen can interrupt conduction in the nerves.
12. Two groups of veins return blood to the heart from the legs.
13. We classify various types of epithelium, mainly according to cell shape.
14. The presence of infection accelerates the flow of lymph.
15. We find sucrose in the sap of many plants.

EXERCISE D *The impersonal use of* it

Verbs of thinking, knowing, speaking, arguing, etc. may be made more impersonal by using *it* + passive verb instead of the personal agent + active verb.

EXAMPLE
  (a) You may see that the study of the nervous system requires a number of histological techniques.
  (b) It may be seen that the study of the nervous system requires a number of histological techniques.

Sentences like example (b) are usually preferred in medical writing, because they are impersonal.

Make the following sentences impersonal in the same way.

1. Students should note that phase-contrast microscopy is not useful with fixed and stained material.
2. You may readily appreciate that a polarizing microscope is particularly valuable when used in conjunction with histochemical methods.
3. I may conclude that the increase in oxygen consumption during exercise depends partly on the increase of metabolic products.
4. Researchers have shown that fluids containing picric acid preserve both tissues and glycogen.
5. Physiologists now think that the blood sugar concentration is controlled by a centre in the fore-brain.
6. You will observe that oxygen is never wholly removed from the blood.
7. They have pointed out that apnoea occurs when connections between the pontine and medullary centres are cut.
8. You must remember that glycogen is generally soluble in water.

EXERCISE E *Nouns formed from verbs*

In the following sentences, change the verbs in italics to their related nouns. Make the other necessary changes in the sentences. Sometimes additional material is provided in brackets at the end of the sentence to help you.

EXAMPLES
(a) When we *study* cell structure we are limited by the techniques available.
The *study* of cell structure is limited by the techniques available.
(b) We could not *investigate* the ribosomes until the EM was *developed*. (had to wait)
The investigation of the ribosomes had to await the development of the EM.

1. An apochromatic lens is *used* to eliminate colour aberrations.
2. As methods of light microscopy *improved*, we *understood* more about cell structure. (increased)
3. Even weak visible fluorescence is adequate if we are *examining* microscopically.
4. Small amounts of fluorescent dye can be *added* to living cells without *damaging* them. (cause)
5. In order to *demonstrate* reticulin fibres properly, metallic impregnation methods are necessary.
6. DNA is *reproduced* during cellular division. (occurs)
7. The fluorescent acridine orange technique was *discovered* accidentally.
8. Formalin pigment is *produced* as a result of tissue fixation. (cause)
9. An optical microscope has the power of *magnifying* up to 1,000 times.
10. You may require a very fine needle to *remove* a specimen.

III INFORMATION TRANSFER

1. Use the diagram to complete the following paragraph. Write the paragraph in your notebook.

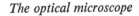

The optical microscope

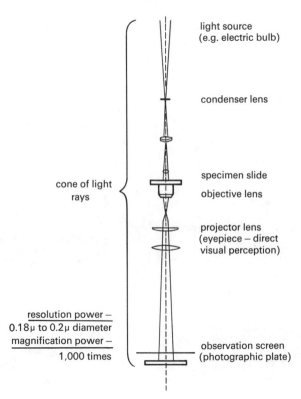

light source
(e.g. electric bulb)

condenser lens

specimen slide
objective lens

projector lens
(eyepiece – direct
visual perception)

cone of light
rays

resolution power –
0.18μ to 0.2μ diameter
magnification power –
1,000 times

observation screen
(photographic plate)

In an ...... microscope a ...... is projected from a source such as an ...... This cone is focused by a ...... on the ...... An ...... magnifies the specimen and projects it into a ...... or ...... At this point ...... is possible. It is also possible for the magnified image of the specimen to be viewed on an ...... or a ...... Although a very useful tool for the study of living tissue, the ...... has a ...... only of particles ...... in diameter. The ...... of the ...... is not greater than ...... times.

2. Use the diagram to complete the following paragraph. Write the paragraph in your notebook.

The electron microscope

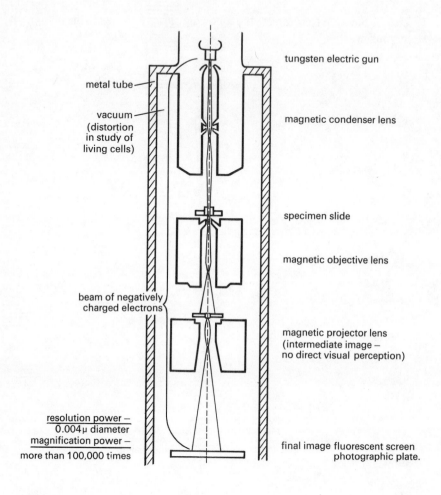

In an ...... microscope a beam of ...... is projected by a ...... This beam is focused on ...... by ...... Beneath the slide is ...... which magnifies the ...... and projects it into ...... Here an ...... image is formed, but no ..... is possible with the EM. The ...... appears only on ...... screen or ...... Because the ...... is enclosed in ...... to create a ......, the study of ...... is subject to ...... Nevertheless ...... is an extremely valuable tool with ...... for particles with a diameter to ...... and ...... to ...... times.

3. Copy the following table into your notebook, using the information in sections 1 and 2 above to complete it.

	Major differences between the optical microscope and the electron microscope	
medium	a cone of light rays	
types of perception possible	(a) the naked eye (b) (c)	(a) (b)
study of living cells	no distortion	
resolution power		
magnification power		

4. Write a brief paragraph describing differences between the optical microscope and the electron microscope.

IV GUIDED WRITING

STAGE 1 *Sentence building*

Join each of the groups of sentences below into one longer sentence, using the additional words printed in capital letters above some of the groups. Omit and replace words as necessary.

1. CAN BE MADE/BETWEEN/AND
   We can make a further distinction.
   We can distinguish desoxyribo-nucleic acid.
   We can also distinguish ribo-nucleic acid.

2. IT IS SAID/THE/OF
   We say that these acids have a special property.
   This property is called basophilia.

3. IS THE STUDY OF/AND
   In histochemistry we study the chemical constituents of cells and tissues.
   We study their distribution.
   We study their function.

4. CAN BE TRACED/BY/WHILE/TO
   We can trace desoxyribo-nucleic acid.
   The Feulgen Method is used.
   Ribo-nucleic acid reacts.
   An enzyme is used.

5. There are acid substances in the nucleus of a cell.
   These attract basic dyes.

6. CAN BE USED/TO/AND
   Spectographic methods are useful.
   They determine the quantity of chemicals.
   They determine changes in their distribution.
   These changes occur during cell activity.

7. THE USE OF
   Histochemistry depends on particular kinds of stains.
   These are selective stains.

8. AND/PROVIDE
   Chemists study rates of absorption and solubility.
   They study actual chemical combination.
   These facts are valuable data.

STAGE 2 *Paragraph building*

Rewrite the eight completed sentences in a logical order to make a paragraph, making the following changes to the sentences indicated:

   write 'the former' for 'desoxyribo-nucleic acid' in sentence 4
   write 'the latter' for 'ribo-nucleic acid' in sentence 4
   add 'for example' to sentence 5
   write 'these chemicals' for 'chemicals' in sentence 6
   write 'it' for 'histochemistry' in sentence 7
   add 'in large part' to sentence 7.

When you have written your paragraph, re-read it and make sure the sentences are presented in a logical order. Give the paragraph a suitable title. Compare your paragraph with the relevant paragraph in the Free Reading section. Make any changes that you think are necessary but remember that sentences can often be arranged in more than one way.

STAGE 3 *Paragraph reconstruction*

Read through the paragraph again. Make sure you know all the words, using a dictionary if necessary. Without referring to your previous work, rewrite the paragraph. Here are some notes to help you.

histochemistry – study of – chemical constituents – cells and tissues – distribution – function
histochemistry – depends – selective stains
acid substances – nucleus of cell – attract basic dyes
these acids – property – basophilia
desoxyribo-nucleic acid – ribo-nucleic acid
former – Feulgen Method – latter – enzyme
spectographic methods – quantity of chemicals – changes in distribution – during cell activity
rates of absorption – solubility – chemical combination – valuable data

V FREE READING

Read the following passage in your own time. Try to find additional examples of the points you have studied in this and other units.

Techniques in the Study of Cell Structure

Microscopic anatomy can be divided into two main parts: the study of tissues taken after death and the study *in vivo* or *in vitro* of living tissues. In the study of tissues taken after death the use of stains is of fundamental importance. Because particular types of cells and structures within the cells attract particular dyes, the physical characteristics of many cellular elements are easily differentiated. Structures which are invisible because their refractility equals that of their surrounding medium may often be defined by staining.

Histochemistry is the study of the chemical constituents of cells and tissues, their distribution and function. It depends in large part on the use of selective stains. For example, acid substances in the nucleus of a cell attract basic dyes. It is said that these acids have the property of basophilia. A further distinction can be made between desoxyribo-nucleic acid and ribonucleic acid. The former can be traced by the Feulgen Method, while the latter reacts to an enzyme. Spectrographic methods can be used to determine the quantity of these chemicals and changes in their distribution during cell activity. Rates of absorption, solubility and actual chemical combination provide valuable data.

In addition to selective staining, it is possible to study certain tissues with the help of metallic salts. Some elements attract deposits of these salts, but since many reagents act both by staining and by impregnation with deposits, it is difficult to separate the two processes.

Tissues fixed and stained after death are usually studied in the form of film preparations or sections. The specimen is frozen or sealed in paraffin or celloidin. A microtome is used to cut the extremely thin sections required for microscopic examination. The preparation of a microscopic section necessarily involves some distortion of the cell from its living counterpart.

Histological techniques involved in the investigation of the detailed anatomy of organs and tissues and especially of embryonic development often depend on the use of serial sections and enlarged models reconstructed from the sections. Serial sections can be prepared of embryos at different stages of development. Each series of sections records one particular phase. When placed in order the series shows the progressive elaboration of an embryo at different ages. Large scale models can then be made of each section and these fitted together to give a three-dimensional reconstruction of the embryo.

The study of tissues *in vivo* is the direct examination of living cells *in situ* by special optical methods. The translucent organs of amphibians and larvae have been extensively studied of late, as have the fluids and cellular structures visible through the membranes of anaesthetized animals. It is also possible today to construct a viewing chamber using thin plates of mica or plastic secured to test animals. Non-toxic dyes can be injected as an aid to examination and such a chamber can be observed over considerable periods of time. Since cells and tissues are in a state of continual activity and change, the value of such observations of living processes cannot be overestimated.

Considerable advances in culture technique have increased the importance of the study of tissues *in vitro*. Fresh tissue is placed in a suitable nutrient material and then aseptically sealed. Successful cell culture depends on an acceptable nutrient, careful temperature control, frequent cleansing away of metabolites, and growth stimulation by feeding embryonic extracts. Examination *in vitro* is particularly valuable for muscle, nerve and epithelial tissue. It is also possible to cultivate embryonic forms of whole organs such as the eye and the internal ear.

6 The Heart

---

[1]The heart is a hollow, cone-shaped organ. [2] It is about the size of a fist and weighs approximately 230g. [3]The base of the heart, which is directed backwards, lies opposite the borders of the 5th, 6th, 7th and 8th thoracic vertebrae. [4]The apex is directed forwards, downwards, and to the left, and is located below the 5th left intercostal space in the mid-clavicular line. [5]In addition to the base and the apex, three surfaces are usually described: the sterno-costal, the left and the diaphragmatic. [6]The sterno-costal surface is limited by four borders, which are sometimes referred to as the borders of the heart.

(a) The heart lies opposite the borders of the 5th, 6th, 7th and 8th thoracic vertebrae.
(b) The apex of the heart lies above the base.
(c) the borders of the heart = the borders of the sterno-costal surface

[7]The heart is essentially a hollow muscle. [8]The wall of the heart is made up of three layers of tissue. [9]A serous membrane, the pericardium, forms the outer covering of the heart. [10]The middle layer, the myocardium, is the heart muscle proper. [11]This consists of specialized cardiac muscle fibres. [12]Internally the heart is lined throughout with a serous membrane known as the endocardium.

[13]The cavity of the heart is divided longitudinally into two parts by a thick septum. [14]Each side contains two chambers: a posterior chamber called the atrium, where the blood is received from the veins and collected, and a thickly muscled anterior chamber called the ventricle, which pumps the blood out again into the arteries. [15]The atria lie above the ventricles. [16]The base of the heart is formed mainly by the left atrium, and partly by the right atrium. [17]The apex is formed entirely by the left ventricle.

(d) The wall of the heart consists mainly of specialized cardiac muscle fibres.
(e) A vertical septum divides the heart.
(f) The heart contains four chambers.
(g) The ventricles lie inferior to the atria.

[18]The heart pumps blood round two circuits: the pulmonary and the systemic. [19]Blood flows into the right atrium from the superior and inferior venae cavae. [20]It passes into the right ventricle, which pumps it out along the pulmonary artery to the lungs. [21]There it is cleansed of carbon dioxide and re-oxygenated. [22]It returns along the pulmonary veins to the left atrium, passes into the left ventricle, and is pumped out into the aorta.

(h)   The right ventricle pumps blood round the pulmonary circuit.
(i)   The right atrium receives blood from the pulmonary circuit.
(j)   Blood always enters the heart by veins and leaves the heart through arteries.

[23]The pumping action of the heart is effected by rhythmic contraction of the muscle, and valves ensure that the blood is propelled in the right direction. [24]The atria are separated from the ventricles by valves which allow the blood to pass freely from the atria into the ventricles, but prevent the blood from returning into the atria when the ventricles contract. [25]These valves are formed by flaps of endocardium which hang down into the ventricles. [26]When the ventricles are full of blood, the blood pushes the flaps upwards to close the orifice. [27]The right atrio-ventricular orifice is closed by three flaps, known as the tricuspid valve. [28]The mitral valve, which consists of two flaps, closes the left atrio-ventricular orifice. [29]The semi-lunar valves, so called because of the half-moon shape of the flaps, lie at the exits of the ventricles, one between the right ventricle and the pulmonary artery, and one between the left ventricle and the aorta. [30]These valves too prevent the reflux of blood and help to maintain the pressure necessary for circulation. [31]When the blood pressure in the arteries exceeds the blood pressure in the ventricles, the flaps of the semi-lunar valves close.

(k)   The atrio-ventricular valves help to retain blood in the atria.
(l)   There are three valves in the right atrio-ventricular orifice.
(m)   The mitral valve is composed of a serous membrane.
(n)   The semi-lunar valves prevent the blood pressure in the arteries from exceeding the blood pressure in the ventricles.

Solutions

(a)   The base of the heart ... lies opposite the borders of the 5th, 6th, 7th and 8th thoracic vertebrae. (3)
the base of the heart ≠ the heart
∴   It is NOT TRUE that the heart lies opposite the borders of the 5th, 6th, 7th and 8th thoracic vertebrae.

(b)   The apex is directed ... downwards. (4)
i.e.   The apex lies below the base.
∴   It is NOT TRUE that the apex of the heart lies above the base.

(c) The sterno-costal surface is limited by four borders, which are sometimes referred to as the borders of the heart. (6)

∴ *the borders of the heart = the borders of the sterno-costal surface*

(d) The heart is essentially a hollow muscle. (7)

i.e. The wall of the heart consists mainly of muscle.
The middle layer, the myocardium, is the heart muscle proper. (10)
This consists of specialized cardiac muscle fibres. (11)

∴ *The wall of the heart consists mainly of specialized cardiac muscle fibres.*

(e) The cavity of the heart is divided longitudinally ... by a thick septum. (13)

longitudinally = from bottom to top of the organ
vertically = from bottom to top, with relation to the anatomical position (see Unit 3)

i.e. longitudinally ≠ vertically

∴ It is NOT TRUE that a vertical septum divides the heart.

(f) The cavity of the heart is divided ... into two parts. (13)
Each side (= each part) contains two chambers. (14)

∴ *The heart contains four chambers.*

(g) The atria lie above the ventricles. (15)

∴ The ventricles lie BELOW the atria.

i.e. *The ventricles lie inferior to the atria.*

(h) The right ventricle ... pumps it (blood) out along the pulmonary artery to the lungs. (20)

i.e. *The right ventricle pumps blood round the pulmonary circuit.*

(i) It (blood) returns along the pulmonary veins to the left atrium. (22)

i.e. The LEFT atrium receives blood from the pulmonary circuit.

∴ It is NOT TRUE that the right atrium receives blood from the pulmonary circuit. (The right atrium receives blood from the venae cavae.) (see 19)

(j) Blood enters the right atrium by veins (the superior and inferior venae cavae). (see 19)
Blood enters the left atrium by veins (the pulmonary veins). (see 22)
Blood leaves the right ventricle by an artery (the pulmonary artery). (see 20)
Blood leaves the left ventricle by an artery (the aorta). (see 22). See also (14)

i.e. *Blood always enters the heart by veins and leaves the heart through arteries.*

(k) The atria are separated from the ventricles by valves which allow the blood to pass freely from the atria into the ventricles. (24)

i.e. The atrio-ventricular valves allow blood to pass freely from the atria.

∴   It is NOT TRUE that the atrio-ventricular valves help to retain blood in the atria.

(l) The right atrio-ventricular orifice is closed by three flaps, known as the tricuspid valve. (27)

     the three flaps = the tricuspid valve

i.e. There are three FLAPS, or one VALVE, in the right atrio-ventricular orifice.

∴   It is NOT TRUE that there are three valves in the right atrio-ventricular orifice.

(m) The mitral valve ... consists of two flaps. (28)

     The valves are formed by flaps of endocardium. (25)

     a serous membrane known as the endocardium (12)

i.e. The mitral valve is composed of endocardium, which is a serous membrane.

∴   *The mitral valve is composed of a serous membrane.*

(n) When the blood pressure in the arteries exceeds the blood pressure in the ventricles, the flaps of the semi-lunar valves close. (31)

i.e. The semi-lunar valves close JUST AFTER the blood pressure in the arteries exceeds the blood pressure in the ventricles.

∴   It is NOT TRUE that the semi-lunar valves prevent the blood pressure in the arteries from exceeding the blood pressure in the ventricles.

EXERCISE A *Contextual reference*

Write the following sentences in your notebook, and complete them after studying the reading passage.
1. 'which' in sentence 3 refers to ......
2. 'which' in sentence 20 refers to ......
3. 'it' in sentence 22 refers to ......
4. 'these valves' in sentence 25 refers to ......
5. 'one' in sentence 29 refers to ......
6. 'these valves' in sentence 30 refers to ......

EXERCISE B *Rephrasing*

Rewrite the following sentences, replacing the words printed in italics with expressions from the reading passage which have the same meaning.
1. The heart *is situated* between the lungs.
2. The sinu-atrial node initiates *heart* action.

3. The heart muscle proper is *referred to as* the myocardium.
4. The endocardium lines the inside of the heart *completely*.
5. Blood *flows* along the pulmonary artery to the lungs.
6. Blood is *purified* in the *lung* capillaries.
7. The oxygenated blood *enters* the left atrium.
8. Blood in the contracting ventricle *forces* upwards the flaps of the tricuspid valve.
9. The *arterial valves* close when the pressure in the arteries *is greater than* the pressure in the ventricles.
10. The mitral valve prevents the *return* of blood into the left atrium.

EXERCISE C *Relationships between statements*

Place the following expressions in the sentences indicated, making any changes necessary.

(a) it should be noted that (5)   (d) then (20)
(b) in fact (16)   (e) then (22)
(c) on the other hand (17)   (f) for (31)

II USE OF LANGUAGE

EXERCISE A pass, flow *and prepositions*

(a) Copy the diagram below into your notebook. Refer to the reading passage and complete the labelling of the diagram by filling in the blanks.
In addition, mark the left atrium (L.A.), right ventricle (R.V.), left ventricle (L.V.), the base, the apex and the septum. The right atrium (R.A.) has been already marked, as an example.

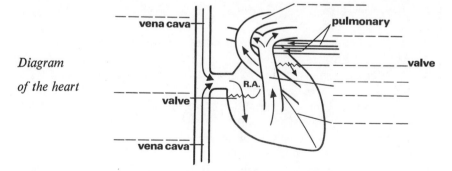

Diagram of the heart

NOTE The arrows indicate the direction of blood flow.

(b) Write out the sentences below, completing them with reference to the diagram. Use the verbs *pass* or *flow*, and appropriate prepositions.

1. Blood ...... from the venae cavae into the ......
2. Blood ...... through the ...... the right ventricle.
3. Blood ...... out of the ...... the pulmonary artery.
4. It ...... the pulmonary artery ...... the lungs.
5. It returns ...... the lungs ...... the pulmonary ...... the left ......
6. It ...... valve ...... the left ventricle, which pumps it out ......

EXERCISE B *The use of time expressions* (i)

Different time expressions can be used to give the same meaning.

EXAMPLE
    Blood fills the ventricle. *Then* the valve closes. (time adverbial)
= *After* blood fills the ventricle, the valve closes. (time conjunction)
= Blood fills the ventricle *before* the valve closes. (time conjunction)

   Join each of the following pairs of sentences into a single sentence with the same meaning. Omit the time adverbial in italics, and choose a suitable time conjunction from the brackets at the end of the sentences.

EXAMPLE
    Blood is pumped out by the left ventricle. *Then* it is carried to all parts of the body. (while, after)
= *After* blood is pumped out by the left ventricle, it is carried to all parts of the body.

1. Food is converted in the stomach to chyme. *Then* it passes through the pyloric sphincter into the duodenum. (after, until)
2. Food remains in the stomach. *After some time* it becomes chyme. (when, until)
3. Blood passes into the right atrium. *Next* it flows into the right ventricle. (before, as)
4. The lungs fill with air. *At the same time* the diaphragm descends and the thorax expands. (as soon as, until)
5. The blood is *first* reoxygenated and cleansed of carbon dioxide. *Then* it returns to the heart. (while, after)
6. Fat is absorbed through the wall of the intestine. *Afterwards* it is carried away in the lymph. (after, until)
7. The glucose is converted into glycogen. *After that* it remains in the liver until it is required. (after, until)
8. Food passes down the oesophagus in the form of a bolus. *At the same time* the oesophagus expands. (as, before)

9. The acid chyme is made more alkaline in the duodenum. *During this process* the pyloric sphincter remains closed. (after, while)
10. Arterial pressure exceeds ventricular pressure. *Immediately* the semi-lunar valves close. (before, as soon as)

EXERCISE C *The use of time expressions* (ii)

Compare the following sentences with the sentences in Exercise B. In each case, write 'same meaning' or 'different meaning' in your notebook.

EXAMPLE

Blood is pumped out by the left ventricle as soon as it is carried to all parts of the body.—different meaning.

1. Food is converted in the stomach to chyme before it passes through the pyloric sphincter into the duodenum.
2. Food becomes chyme and remains in the stomach.
3. Before blood passes into the right atrium, it flows into the right ventricle.
4. The lungs fill with air, and simultaneously the diaphragm descends and the thorax expands.
5. Blood returns to the heart and then it is reoxygenated and cleansed of carbon dioxide.
6. As soon as fat is carried away in the lymph, it is absorbed through the wall of the intestine.
7. The glucose is converted into glycogen and it remains in the liver until it is required.
8. After the oesophagus expands, food passes down it in the form of a bolus.
9. The pyloric sphincter remains closed while the acid chyme is made more alkaline in the duodenum.
10. When arterial pressure exceeds ventricular pressure, the semi-lunar valves close.

EXERCISE D *Listing* (ii)

In medical writing, the following is a very common sentence pattern:
    There are X parts: a, b, c, and d.

EXAMPLES

(a) There are *four* valves in the heart: the mitral valve, the tricuspid valve, the pulmonary valve and the aortic valve.
(b) The heart pumps blood round *two* circuits: the pulmonary and the systemic.

(c) Each side of the heart contains *two* chambers: a posterior thin-walled chamber called the atrium, and an anterior chamber which is more thickly muscled and is known as the ventricle.

Notice that in this sentence pattern

(i) the first part of the sentence contains a number; this is the number of items listed in the second part of the sentence.
(ii) the first part of the sentence is divided from the second part by a colon.
(iii) the second part of the sentence (i.e. the list) contains no main clause. Items may be qualified: e.g. by adjectives, relative clauses or short-form relative clauses.

Make each of the following short paragraphs into a sentence of the pattern illustrated above. Fill in the number and use a colon. Make any changes necessary, so that there are no main clauses within the list.

EXAMPLE
The skin consists of ... layers. The epidermis, or surface layer, is composed of epithelial tissue. The dermis, or deeper layer, is composed of connective tissue.
= The skin consists of two layers: the epidermis, or surface layer, composed of epithelial tissue, and the dermis, or deeper layer, which is composed of connective tissue.

NOTE
If items seem very long, they may be separated by semi-colons instead of commas.

1. The heart is divided into ... cavities. These are the right atrium, the right ventricle, the left atrium and the left ventricle.
2. The adrenal glands consist of ... parts. These are the outer part, or cortex, and the inner part, or medulla.
3. The heart is usually considered to have ... surfaces. These are the sternocostal surface, the left surface, and the diaphragmatic surface.
4. The oesophagus is made up of ... layers of tissue. There is an inner mucous coat. Next there is a submucous coat which contains large blood vessels and nerves. Then there is a layer of muscle. Finally there is a coat of fibrous connective tissue.
5. The stomach consists of ... parts. There is a large vertical portion on the left. A smaller transverse portion lies below it and to the right.
6. ... layers of tissue form the heart wall. A serous membrane, known as the pericardium, forms the outer surface. The myocardium or heart muscle makes up the main part of the wall. The endocardium, another serous membrane, forms the inner surface.

7. The normal skeleton is made up of ... bones. There are 86 pairs of bones. In addition, there are 34 single bones.
8. There are ... kinds of tongue papillae. The filiform papillae are found all over the tongue. The fungiform papillae lie on the top and side of the tongue. The circumvallate papillae are situated at the base of the tongue.
9. The heart is supplied with ... sets of nerve fibres. One set runs from the medulla oblongata in the vagus nerve. The second set runs from the sympathetic ganglion at the base of the neck.
10. There are ... pairs of salivary glands. The parotid glands are in front of each ear. The submaxillary glands are beneath the mandible. The sublingual glands lie beneath the tongue.
11. The stomach wall consists of ... coats. There is an outer serous lining known as the peritoneum. Next is a coat of muscle fibres, and then a submucous coat. The submucous coat connects the muscular layer to the innermost layer, which is a thick coat of mucus.
12. There are ... types of muscular tissue. Plain muscle is the simplest kind. It is found in the walls of hollow viscera and of blood vessels. Striated muscle is composed of more specialized fibres. These are usually arranged in bundles. Cardiac muscle is structurally intermediate between plain muscle and striated muscle.

EXERCISE E *Compound adjectives*

An important feature of medical terminology is the compound adjective made up from two nouns. The first part usually ends in *-o* and the second part has an adjectival ending.

EXAMPLES
> the *atrio-ventricular* valves (atrium + ventricle)
> the *coraco-acromial* arch (coracoid process + acromion)
> the *tracheo-bronchial* lymph glands (trachea + bronchi)

Both parts of the compound adjective must be derived from Latin or Greek. Notice that the nouns in the brackets above are all directly derived from Latin or Greek. When the noun is not directly derived from Latin or Greek (e.g. rib, liver) then the corresponding Latin or Greek stem must be used to make up the adjective.

EXAMPLES
> the *costo-diaphragmatic* recess (rib + diaphragm)
>   rib: Lat. cost-
> the *hepato-colic* ligament (liver + colon)
>   liver: Gr. hepat-

Write out the following sentences, completing the compound adjective in each case.

1. The surface facing the sternum and ribs is known as the . . . -costal surface.
2. The joint between the acromion and the clavicle is called the . . . -clavicular joint.
3. The joint between the sternum and the clavicle is called the . . . joint.
4. The ligament between the ribs and the clavicle is called the . . . ligament. (*rib:* Lat. *cost-*)
5. The pouch between the rectum and the uterus is referred to as the . . . -uterine pouch.
6. The valve between the ileum and the colon is known as the . . . -colic valve.
7. The fold round the stomach and the pancreas is called the . . . -pancreatic fold. (*stomach:* Gr. *gastr-*)
8. The flexure made by the duodenum and the jejunum is known as the . . . -jejunal flexure.
9. The joint between the sacrum and the ilium is referred to as the . . . -iliac joint.
10. The joints between the carpals and the metacarpals are known as the . . . -metacarpal joints.
11. The joints between the tarsals and the metatarsals are known as the . . . joints.
12. The cavity of the nose and the pharynx is named the . . . -pharyngeal cavity. (*nose:* Lat. *nas-*)
13. The nerve supplying the tongue and the pharynx is known as the . . . nerve. (*tongue:* Gr. *gloss-*)
14. The fascia of the cheek and the pharynx is referred to as the . . . fascia. (*cheek:* Lat. *bucc-*)
15. The joint between the sacrum and the coccyx is called the . . . -coccygeal joint.
16. The joint between the radius and the ulna is known as the . . . -ulnar joint.
17. The junction of the ileum and the caecum is called the . . . -caecal junction.
18. The opening between the pleura and the peritoneum is known as the . . . -peritoneal opening.
19. The canal between the pericardium and the peritoneum is called the . . . canal.
20. The ligament joining the sternum and the pericardium is known as the . . . -pericardial ligament.
21. The opening between the pleura and the pericardium is known as the . . . opening.
22. The ligaments between the ribs and the pericardium are called the . . . ligaments. (*rib:* Lat. *cost-*)

III INFORMATION TRANSFER

1. Look at the following diagram. Write out the paragraph and complete it
   with reference to the diagram.

Osmosis in a capillary (systemic circuit)

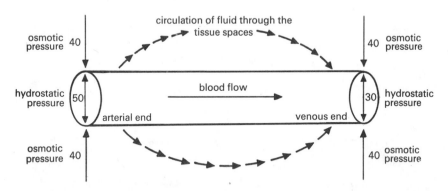

As the blood ...... from the arterial ...... to the ...... of the ......,
the ...... pressure decreases. In this example, it ...... from ...... mm of
mercury to ...... mm. The ......, however, remains constant at ......mm.
At the arterial end, the ...... exceeds the ...... by ...... mm, and so
fluid passes out of the capillary into the ...... At the ...... end, the ......
is less than the ...... by ...... mm, and so approximately the same amount
of ...... passes out of the ...... into the ...... Thus the difference in
pressures causes the ...... through the ......

2. Look at the following diagram. Write out the paragraph and complete it
   with reference to the diagram. The paragraph you have just written in
   section 1 should help you.

Osmosis in a capillary (in oedema)

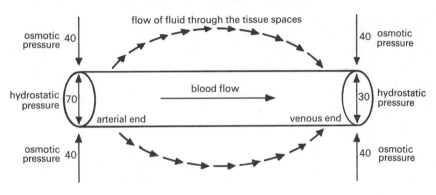

As the blood ...... from ...... to ...... of ......, the hydrostatic pressure ...... In this example, it ...... The ......, however, remains ...... 40 mm. At the ......, the hydrostatic pressure ...... by ...... and so fluid ...... At the ......, the hydrostatic pressure ...... by ......, and so a smaller amount of fluid returns to the ...... Thus excess fluid collects in the ......

3. Look at the following diagram and write a paragraph showing how osmosis in a pulmonary capillary keeps the tissue of the lungs free from fluid. The paragraphs you have just written in sections 1 and 2 should help you.

Osmosis in a capillary (pulmonary circuit)

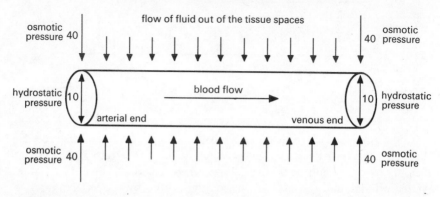

As ......, the hydrostatic pressure ...... constant at ...... mercury. The osmotic pressure ...... The osmotic pressure ...... the hydrostatic pressure all along the capillary, and so ...... passes out of the ...... No fluid returns ...... Thus the tissue of the lungs is kept free from ......

4. Look at the following diagram and write a paragraph showing how in left ventricular failure the tissue of the lungs becomes saturated in fluid.

Osmosis in a pulmonary capillary (in left ventricular failure)

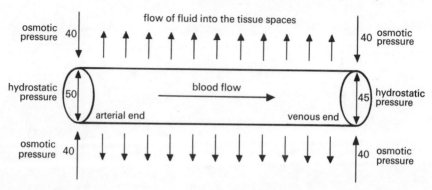

IV GUIDED WRITING

STAGE 1 *Sentence and paragraph building*

Make a paragraph from the following list of short sentences. You may retain some sentences as they are; other sentences may be joined together using *therefore, when, until* or *as.* Your paragraph should contain about 16 sentences.

The sentences are already in a logical order, but you may want to change the order when you are combining them.

A complete heart beat lasts approximately 0·8 second.
For about 0·4 second the heart is relaxed.
This is known as the period of diastole.
During the period of diastole the atrio-ventricular valves are open.
The arterial valves are closed.
The heart fills with blood.
At the same time the heart expands from its previous contraction.
Blood flows into the two atria.
It flows through the open atrio-ventricular valves.
It flows into the two ventricles.
Then the period of systole begins.
The atria both contract.
They force more blood into the ventricles.
The phase of atrial systole lasts about 0·1 second.
The impulse to contract is conducted along the bundle of His to the ventricles.
The period of ventricular systole begins.
It lasts about 0·3 second.
The ventricles begin to contract.
The atrio-ventricular valves are closed by the upward movement of the blood.
The ventricular pressure rises.
The ventricular pressure is greater than the pressure in the aorta and the pulmonary artery.
Then the arterial valves open.
The contraction continues.
Blood is ejected from the ventricles into the arteries.
At the end of the period of systole, the ventricles begin to relax.
The ventricular pressure drops below the arterial pressure.
The arterial valves close.
Almost immediately the ventricular pressure becomes less than the atrial pressure.
The atrio-ventricular valves open.
The period of diastole begins again.

Re-read your paragraph and make sure it is coherent. Then check it with the relevant paragraph in the Free Reading section. Remember that more than one version is possible.

STAGE 2 *Paragraph reconstruction*

Read through your paragraph again. Make sure you know all the words, using a dictionary if necessary. Without referring to your previous work, rewrite the paragraph. Here are some notes to help you.

heart beat
0·8 second

diastole
0·4 second – heart relaxed
atrio-ventricular valves open – arterial valves closed
heart fills with blood – expands
blood flows into two atria – through atrio-ventricular valves – into two
    ventricles

systole
(*a*) *atrial systole*
both atria contract – more blood into ventricles
0·1 second
impulse to contract – bundle of His – ventricles

(*b*) *ventricular systole*
0·3 second
both ventricles contract – atrio-ventricular valves – closed by blood
ventricular pressure – greater – pressure in aorta and pulmonary artery
arterial valves open – blood ejected
ventricles relax – ventricular pressure drops – arterial valves close
ventricular pressure – atrial pressure – atrio-ventricular valves open

diastole
begins again

V   FREE READING

Read the following passage in your own time. Try to find additional examples of the points you have studied in this and other units.

Heart Action

The contraction and relaxation of the heart is called the heart beat. The heart beat is myogenic, i.e. it is an inherent property of heart muscle, not dependent on the central nervous system. This has been demonstrated in various ways. For example, strips of cardiac muscle containing no nervous tissue will beat indefinitely when immersed in a solution of certain salts. It has also been shown that a chick embryo heart begins to beat before it is innervated.

Certain parts of the myocardium have the special function of controlling heart action. A small collection of these specialized cardiac muscle fibres, known as the sinu-atrial node, is found in the wall of the right atrium, near the entrance of the venae cavae. The sinu-atrial node acts as a pacemaker, initiating the phase of contraction and controlling its regularity. Another collection of specialized heart muscle, often referred to as the bundle of His, passes from the septal wall of the right atrium down the septum into both ventricles, transmitting to the ventricles the impulse from the atrium. Thus the rhythm of ventricular contraction is made to follow the rhythm of atrial contraction.

A complete heart beat lasts approximately 0·8 second. For about 0·4 second the heart is relaxed. This is known as the period of diastole. During the period of diastole, the atrio-ventricular valves are open and the arterial valves are closed. The heart therefore fills with blood at the same time as it expands from its previous contraction. Blood flows into the two atria and through the open atrio-ventricular valves into the two ventricles. Then the period of systole begins. The atria both contract, forcing more blood into the ventricles. The phase of atrial systole lasts about 0·1 second. The impulse to contract is conducted along the bundle of His to the ventricles and the period of ventricular systole, lasting about 0·3 second, begins. When the ventricles begin to contract, the atrio-ventricular valves are closed by the upward movement of the blood. The ventricular pressure rises until it is greater than the pressure in the aorta and the pulmonary artery. Then the arterial valves open and, as the contraction continues, blood is ejected from the ventricles into the arteries. At the end of the period of systole, the ventricles begin to relax, the ventricular pressure drops below the arterial pressure, and the arterial valves close. Almost immediately the ventricular pressure becomes less than the atrial pressure, the atrio-ventricular valves open, and the period of diastole begins again.

Since all of the blood goes round both the pulmonary and the systemic circuits, the same amount of blood must be pumped out by each ventricle. The volume pumped out by one ventricle at a single beat (the stroke volume) varies from about 70 cc at rest to about 200 cc during exertion. The left ventricle, which propels blood round the whole body, has to pump with much more force than the right ventricle, which sends blood only to the lungs and back. The left ventricle in fact pumps at a pressure of about 120 mm of mercury, while the right ventricle pumps at about 25 mm.

Although the stroke volume does increase during exertion, the volume of blood pumped out per minute is more significantly increased by a faster rate of heart beat. The normal heart rate, with each beat lasting about 0·8 second, is about 70 beats per minute. This can be increased when necessary to about 200 beats per minute, with the result that cardiac output can vary from 5 litres per minute at rest to as much as 40 litres per minute. When the heart rate is increased, it is the diastolic phase in particular which is shortened.

7 The Nervous System

---

[1]The basic unit of the nervous system is the neurone, or nerve cell. [2]It consists of a cell body and its processes. [3]Each neurone has two types of process: a number of short, freely branching fibres called dendrites, and a single process called the axon, which may or may not give off branches along its course. [4]The dendrites convey impulses to the cell body; the axon, which is the main conducting fibre, conveys impulses away from the cell body. [5]The axon varies in length in different kinds of neurone. [6]In a motor neurone it can be very long, running, for example, from a cell body in the spinal cord to a muscle in the foot. [7]Axons of the internuncial neurones, which provide links between other neurones, are often short and difficult to distinguish from the dendrites.

(a) A neurone consists of a cell body, dendrites and an axon.
(b) The axon is a freely branching fibre.
(c) The main conducting fibre of a neurone is very long.
(d) Other neurones can be difficult to distinguish from the dendrites.

[8]An unactivated nerve fibre maintains a state of chemical stability with concentrations of potassium inside and outside the lining membrane in a ratio of 30:1. [9]Thus the nerve fibre at rest is electrically charged. [10]A nerve impulse is a wave of depolarization created by a chemical imbalance. [11]Sodium passes through the membrane, releasing potassium. [12]The depolarization of any part of the nerve cell causes the depolarization of the next segment, and so on to the end of the fibre. [13]The end of a nerve fibre is not structurally joined to the next cell, but the small gap between them can be bridged chemically. [14]This functional junction is known as a synapse. [15]Not all the chemicals which act as transmitters are known but among the most important are acetyl choline and noradrenaline. [16]Once the synapse has been made, these chemicals are rapidly destroyed by enzymes. [17]The nerve fibre itself recharges within milliseconds.

(e) An unactivated nerve fibre contains thirty times more potassium than its surrounding tissue.
(f) A nerve impulse is a chemical imbalance.
(g) A synapse is a connection which is made over the small gap between the end of a nerve fibre and the next cell.
(h) Acetyl choline is known to transmit impulses.
(i) Transmitters are destroyed by enzymes.

[18]The brain and spine together form the central nervous system. [19]Arising from the central nervous system and supplying all parts of the body are the peripheral nerves, commonly referred to simply as nerves. [20]A nerve is a cord-like structure, usually containing bundles of conducting fibres, which may be sensory or motor.

(j) The peripheral nerves arise from the brain and the spine.
(k) Nerves may contain axons from both sensory and motor neurones.

[21]Twelve pairs of nerves arise from the brain and thirty-one pairs of nerves arise from the spine. [22]These are known as the cranial nerves and the spinal nerves respectively. [23]Of the twelve cranial nerves, five contain both sensory and motor fibres. [24]The most important of these is the vagus, or tenth nerve, which supplies the heart, most of the digestive organs, the pharynx and the larynx. [25]Of the remaining seven pairs of nerves, four contain motor fibres only, and three are entirely sensory. [26]The fourth and sixth nerves, for example, control the movement of the eyeball, and the first nerve records smells.
[27]In contrast, all the spinal nerves contain both sensory and motor fibres. [28]There are eight pairs of cervical nerves, twelve thoracic, five lumbar, five sacral, and one coccygeal. [29]The spinal nerves divide into two branches. [30]The posterior branches serve the muscles and skin of the back of their own region. [31]The anterior branches of the thoracic nerves circle the thorax, supplying the intercostal muscles and the skin. [32]All other anterior branches form plexuses, or networks of nerve fibres, from which nerves pass out to supply the cervical and pelvic regions and the upper and lower limbs. [33]Thus each limb nerve contains fibres from several spinal nerves. [34]The sciatic nerve, which emerges from the sacral plexus to serve the back of the thigh and the leg, contains fibres from five spinal nerves: the fourth and fifth lumbar nerves, and the first, second and third sacral nerves.

(l) Most of the cranial nerves contain both sensory and motor nerve fibres.
(m) The thirty-one pairs of nerves which arise from the spine are known as the cranial nerves and the spinal nerves respectively.
(n) The cranial nerves supply the head and neck only.

Solutions

(a)   It (a neurone) consists of a cell body and its processes. (2)
Each neurone has two types of process: ... dendrites, and ... the axon. (3)

∴   *A neurone consists of a cell body, dendrites and an axon.*

(b)   The axon ... may or may not give off branches. (3)

i.e.   Some axons give off branches and some axons do not.
  a freely branching fibre = a fibre which gives off very many branches, which themselves may give off more branches
  Some axons do not give off branches. (see 3)

∴   The axon is NOT a freely branching fibre.

(c)   The axon ... is the main conducting fibre. (4)
The axon varies in length. (5)
it can be very long (6)
Axons ... are often short. (7)

∴   The main conducting fibre of a neurone is NOT ALWAYS very long.

(d)   Axons ... are often short and difficult to distinguish from the dendrites. (7)

i.e.   It is axons, NOT other neurones, which can be difficult to distinguish from the dendrites.

(e)   In an unactivated nerve fibre, the concentrations of potassium inside and outside are in a ratio of 30:1. (see 8)

i.e.   The concentration of potassium inside is thirty times more than the concentration of potassium outside.

∴   *An unactivated nerve fibre contains thirty times more potassium than its surrounding tissue.*

(f)   A nerve impulse is a wave of depolarization created by a chemical imbalance. (10)

=   A nerve impulse is a wave of depolarization.
  It is CAUSED BY a chemical imbalance.

∴   It is NOT TRUE that a nerve impulse IS a chemical imbalance.

(g)   A synapse is a functional junction. (see 14)
It is the junction between the end of a nerve fibre and the next cell; they are not joined structurally, as there is a small gap between them. (see 13)
They are joined, or connected, chemically. (see 13)

∴   *A synapse is a connection which is made over the small gap between the end of a nerve fibre and the next cell.*

(h) The most important (of the chemicals which act as transmitters) are acetyl choline and noradrenaline. (15)

i.e. Acetyl choline is known to be a transmitter – one of the most important.

∴ *Acetyl choline is known to transmit impulses.*

(i) These chemicals are rapidly destroyed by enzymes. (16)
   these chemicals = the chemicals which act as transmitters (see 15)

∴ *Transmitters are destroyed by enzymes.*

(j) Arising from the central nervous system ... are the peripheral nerves. (19)
   the central nervous system = the brain and the spine (18)
   The peripheral nerves arise from the brain and the spine.

(k) A nerve contains bundles of conducting fibres. (see 20)
   conducting fibres = axons from neurones (see 4)
   A nerve contains bundles of axons from neurones.
   These may be sensory or motor. (see 20)

∴ *Nerves may contain axons from both sensory and motor neurones.*

(l) Of the twelve cranial nerves, five contain both sensory and motor fibres. (23)

∴ It is NOT TRUE that MOST of the cranial nerves contain both sensory and motor fibres.

(m) These are known as the cranial nerves and the spinal nerves respectively. (22)
   these = the twelve pairs of nerves which arise from the brain and the
      thirty-one pairs of nerves which arise from the spine
   RESPECTIVELY indicates that the first group of nerves has the first name
   and the second group of nerves has the second name.

i.e. The twelve pairs of nerves which arise from the brain are known as the cranial nerves, and the thirty-one pairs of nerves which arise from the spine are known as the spinal nerves.

∴ It is NOT TRUE that the thirty-one pairs of nerves which arise from the spine are known as the cranial nerves and the spinal nerves respectively.

(n) The vagus is a cranial nerve which supplies the heart and most of the digestive organs. (see 24, where these = the twelve cranial nerves)

∴ It is NOT TRUE that the cranial nerves supply the head and neck only.

EXERCISE A *Contextual reference*

Write out the following sentences in your notebook, and complete them after studying the reading passage.
1. 'it' in sentence 2 refers to ...
2. 'its' in sentence 2 refers to ...

3. 'it' in sentence 6 refers to ...
4. 'these' in sentence 22 refers to ...
5. 'these' in sentence 24 refers to ...

EXERCISE B *Rephrasing*

Rewrite the following sentences, replacing the words printed in italics with expressions from the reading passage which have the same meaning.
1. About 100,000 sensory fibres *carry* impulses from the eye to the brain.
2. An unactivated nerve fibre is in a state of chemical *equilibrium*.
3. A nerve impulse is *due to* sodium passing through the membrane and releasing potassium.
4. A spinal nerve passes out from the central nervous system through the *space* between two vertebrae.
5. A synapse may be *formed* with more than one internuncial neurone.
6. *After* the chemical transmitters have contacted the next cell, they are destroyed.
7. The vagus *includes* both sensory and motor fibres.
8. The sciatic nerve *serves* the back of the thigh and the leg.
9. The nerve *passes out* from the brachial plexus to supply the upper arm.
10. In the lumbar region, a *network of nerve fibres* is located in the psoas muscle.

EXERCISE C *Relationships between statements*

Place one of the expressions below in each of the sentences indicated. When necessary, replace and re-order the words in the sentences and change the punctuation.

therefore   on the other hand   for example

(7)   (27)   (34)

II USE OF LANGUAGE

EXERCISE A *Listing* (iii)

See Listing (i) Unit 2.
Sometimes a list may occur inside a list.

EXAMPLE
   The sciatic nerve contains fibres from the fourth and fifth lumbar nerves, and the first, second and third sacral nerves.

This list takes the form: a+b, and c, d+e. It may be presented diagram-matically:

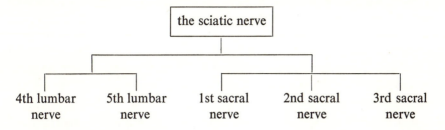

(a) Convert the following diagrams into sentence form, using the example above as a model. The spinal nerves are given their usual notation (i.e. C = cervical, Th = thoracic, L = lumbar, and S = sacral).

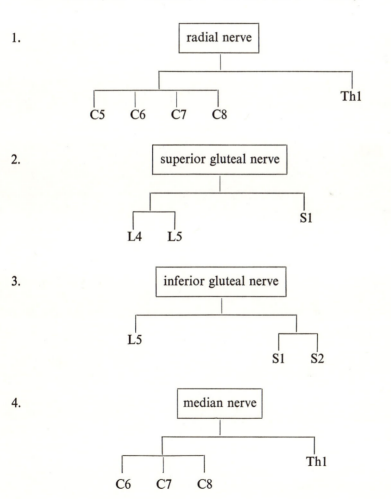

1.

2.

3.

4.

A list is made within a list when the writer wishes to group certain items together. In the examples studied above, spinal nerves were grouped together when they originated from the same region of the spine. Clearly, there may be other reasons for grouping items together.

EXAMPLE
The essentials in the diet are proteins, carbohydrates and fats, mineral salts, and vitamins.

This example takes the form a, b+c, d, and e. The writer has grouped carbohydrates and fats together, because they have a similar function, in providing fuel for the body. (Protein can do this, but it is not its primary function.)

Notice that it would not be wrong to write a plain list with no internal grouping:

EXAMPLE
The essentials in the diet are proteins, carbohydrates, fats, mineral salts, and vitamins.

But often internal grouping can add meaning to a list, making it easier to understand and remember.

(b) Write out the following lists in sentence form.

1. The kidney consists of
    i. the pelvis
    ii. the (a) medulla
          (b) cortex
    iii. an outer capsule of fibrous tissue.
2. The large intestine consists of
    i. the (a) caecum
          (b) vermiform appendix
    ii. the colon
    iii. the rectum
3. The thoracic cavity contains
    i. the (a) lungs
          (b) heart
    ii. the (a) thoracic duct
          (b) other lymph vessels
    iii. blood vessels
    iv. nerves
4. In the female, the pelvic floor supports
    i. the bladder
    ii. the (a) uterus
          (b) vagina
    iii. the rectum

5. The constituents of plasma include
    i. (a) proteins
       (b) amino acids
   ii. fats
  iii. glucose
   iv. (a) urea
      (b) other nitrogenous waste
    v. various salts

EXERCISE B *Combining sentences with an* -ing *clause*

Look at the following sentences:

(a) There is virtually no matrix.
(b) The cells *are situated* almost continuously.

These can be combined into one sentence:

(c) There is virtually no matrix, the cells *being situated* almost continuously.

Look at the following sentences:

(d) The epidermis overlies the dermis.
(e) *It* (the epidermis) *forms* the outer layer of the skin.

These have the same subject. They can be combined into one sentence:

(f) The epidermis overlies the dermis, *forming* the outer layer of the skin.

When the subjects are the same, the subject before the *-ing* form is omitted.

Join each of the following pairs of sentences into one sentence, using the *-ing* form. Remember to omit the subject before the *-ing* form when it is the same as the subject in the main clause.
1. The cephalic vein runs on the lateral side of the forearm and upper arm. The cephalic vein gives off a branch anterior to the elbow to join the basilic vein.
2. The cartilage cells enlarge and arrange themselves in rows. Calcium salts are deposited in the matrix.
3. Blood capillaries accompany the osteoblasts. The blood capillaries ramify in the spaces.
4. The thorax is a very mobile region. The heart and lungs are in rhythmic pulsation.
5. The bladder is emptied from time to time. The urine is expelled to the exterior through a tube called the urethra.
6. On the left side of the thorax anteriorly the breath sounds are more subdued. They are conducted only along the bronchial tree.
7. The alveolar wall is very thin. It consists only of two layers of pavement epithelium.

8. The fibres of the external oblique abdominal muscle radiate downwards and forwards. The lowest fibres pass vertically downwards.
9. Ptyalin begins the digestion of starch. It converts cooked starch into dextrose and maltose.
10. Stratified squamous epithelium consists of layers of cells. The deeper cells have a distinct shape but the more superficial cells are flattened.
11. The cerebral hemispheres fill the top and front portions of the cranial cavity. The cerebral hemispheres stretch from above the foramen magnum to the forehead.
12. The oesophagus extends downwards from the pharynx. It enters the stomach at the cardiac orifice.
13. In the arterioles, which have non-elastic muscular walls, there is a fall in blood pressure. The pressure is used up in overcoming friction.
14. Saliva dissolves part of the food. It makes taste possible.
15. When the amoebic cell reaches adult size, it divides into two daughter cells. The nucleus divides before the rest of the protoplasm.
16. The cells of an epithelium touch one another. There is little or no inter-cellular matrix.
17. Nerve cells have the power of regeneration if the cell body is uninjured. A new axon grows out of the cell body.
18. The sections are de-waxed. Artifact pigments are removed at the same time.
19. Peristalsis is a wave of relaxation followed by a wave of contraction. The circular muscle fibres are inhibited in front of the food and stimulated behind it.
20. The kidneys are 3–4 inches long and $1–1\frac{1}{2}$ inches wide. The left kidney is a little longer and narrower than the right.

EXERCISE C *Short-form time clauses*

Look at the following sentences:

(a) Before *they enter* the heart, the venae cavae fuse.
    Before *entering* the heart, the venae cavae fuse.
(b) When *they are contracted*, the muscles keep the orifice closed.
    When *contracted*, the muscles keep the orifice closed.

The short-form time clause can be used ONLY when the subject of the time-clause is the same as the subject of the main clause.

When the verb in the time clause is active, it is changed to the *-ing* form; when it is passive it is changed to the *-ed* form. (See also short-form relative clauses, Unit 2.) The subject in a short-form time clause is omitted.

Notice that the sentences can also be written:

(a) Before the venae cavae enter the heart, they fuse.
(b) When the muscles are contracted, they keep the orifice closed.

Change the time clauses in the following sentences to short-form time clauses, using the *-ing* or the *-ed* form. Use the same time conjunctions as are in the sentences but notice that *as soon as* should be changed to *on*.

1. When it is examined under a lens, the mucous coat of the stomach presents a honeycombed appearance.
2. After the ileum leaves the pelvic cavity, it passes upwards, backwards, and to the right.
3. The blood distributes heat evenly while it circulates round the body.
4. When the fibres of the diaphragm are relaxed, they curve upwards over the liver, stomach and spleen.
5. Before it ossifies, the sternum is a bar of hyaline cartilage.
6. When the rectum is viewed from the front, it is seen to have three lateral flexures.
7. As soon as it passes through the diaphragm, the thoracic duct enters the posterior mediastinum.
8. The roots of the lumbar and sacral nerves run almost vertically before they leave the spinal canal.
9. When the facial artery passes under the digastric and stylo-hyoid muscles, it comes into contact with the superior constrictor muscle.

EXERCISE D *Inversion*

Look at the following sentences:
(a) The vocal cords stretch across the cavity of the larynx.
(b) Stretching across the cavity of the larynx are the vocal cords.
(c) The sciatic nerve is directed downwards from the sacral plexus.
(d) Directed downwards from the sacral plexus is the sciatic nerve.

(b) and (d) are examples of inversion. Inversion is a common stylistic device in medical writing. It is used when passing from one topic to the next. For example, sentence (b) would be used after a description of the cavity of the larynx, to introduce a description of the vocal cords. Similarly sentence (d) would be used after a description of the sacral plexus, to introduce a description of the sciatic nerve.

Study the example of inversion in the reading passage in Section I of this unit (sentence 19).

When you read the Free Reading section of this unit, notice how inversion is used.

Invert the following sentences.

1. A mucous membrane lines the eyelids.
2. The pleura is reflected back from the lung surface.
3. A crescentic fold is placed at the upper border of the orifice.
4. Little pouches of peritoneum, known as the appendices epiploicae, project from the wall of the large intestine.

5. The sacro-spinous ligament lies on the pelvic surface of the sacro-tuberous ligament.
6. The nerve cells of the sensory neurones are massed together in the ganglia.
7. The darker red cortex surrounds the medulla.
8. The biconvex lens is suspended behind the iris.
9. Delicate protoplasmic threads connect one cell with another.
10. The brachial artery is directed down the upper arm.
11. A layer of flattened cells, called the stratum granulosum, covers the stratum of Malpighi.
12. The common hepatic duct is formed by the union of the right and left hepatic ducts.

III INFORMATION TRANSFER

The Reflex Arc

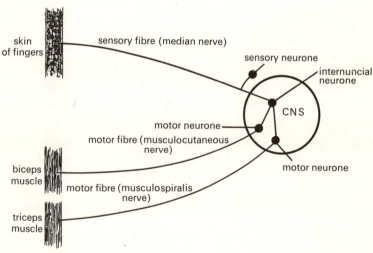

A. A typical reflex arc consists of:

1. stimulation of sensory neurone
2. transmission of impulse along sensory fibre to CNS (central nervous system)
3. synapse with internuncial neurone
4. synapse with motor neurone
5. transmission of impulse along motor fibre to muscle
6. reaction (i.e. relaxation or contraction) of muscle.

B. On page 94 is a simplified diagram of a reflex arc. This reflex arc takes place when the fingers touch something hot and are jerked away from the source of heat by movement of the arm. Use the information given above in A and the information given in the diagram to write an account of this reflex arc. Begin your account: *When the fingers touch something hot, the sensory neurone ....*

IV GUIDED WRITING

STAGE 1 *Sentence building*

Join each of the groups of sentences below into one longer sentence, using the additional words printed in capital letters above some of the groups. Omit words in italics.

1. THIS
   A break in electrical continuity *occurs.*
   It points to some form of non-electrical transmission at the junction.

2. Eserine is added to the frog muscle preparation.
   This addition inhibits the enzyme cholinesterase.
   The enzyme cholinesterase hydrolyses acetylcholine.

3. The transmission is almost certainly by the chemical acetylcholine.
   Other experiments indicate *this.*

4. WHEN
   A microelectrode is placed between the nerve fibre and the muscle cell at the point of junction.
   We can show *this.*
   BEFORE
   The axon potential arrives at the junction.
   The potential is set up in the post-junctional tissue about 0·8 msec *later.*

5. WHEN
   We have shown *this.*
   Acetylcholine is applied by micropipette to the muscle fibre.
   It is applied on the precise point of neuromuscular junction.
   Even minute amounts of acetylcholine can excite the muscle fibre.

6. IF
   The nerve fibre is artificially stimulated.
   An increasing amount of acetylcholine is released from the end of the fibre.

7. Acetylcholine is applied elsewhere on the muscle.
   No response is detected.

STAGE 2 *Paragraph building*

Add the following material to the sentences indicated:

write 'for example' at the beginning of sentence 2
add 'also' to sentence 5
add 'then' to sentence 6
add 'however' to sentence 7.

Rewrite the seven completed sentences in a logical order to make a paragraph. Make sentence 4 the first sentence of the paragraph.

When you have written your paragraph, re-read it and make sure that the sentences are in a logical order. Give your paragraph a suitable title. Compare your paragraph with the relevant paragraph in the Free Reading section. Make any changes that you think are necessary but remember that sentences can often be arranged in more than one way.

STAGE 3 *Paragraph reconstruction*

Read through the paragraph again. Make sure you know all the words, using a dictionary if necessary. Without referring to your previous work, rewrite the paragraph. Here are some notes to help you.

microelectrode – between nerve fibre and muscle cell – point of junction – axon potential – about 0·8 msec before potential in post-junctional tissue
this break in electrical continuity points to – non-electrical transmission – junction
other experiments indicate – transmission – by acetylcholine
add eserine – frog muscle – inhibits cholinesterase – hydrolyses acetylcholine
nerve fibre – artificially stimulated – acetylcholine released
acetylcholine – applied to muscle fibre – neuromuscular junction – excite muscle fibre
applied elsewhere – no response

V   FREE READING

Read the following passage in your own time. Try to find additional examples of the points you have studied in this and other units.

Chemical Transmission in the Nervous System

The electron microscope has shown that a space separates the end of an axon from the cell to which the impulse is transmitted. As the space presumably has the same electrical properties as the axon, the potential cannot cross the gap directly. Instead, when the nerve fibre ending is depolarized, a chemical substance is liberated from the vesicles at the end of the fibre. This substance crosses the gap and alters the permeability of the post-junctional cell membrane, thus initiating another potential.

There is a certain amount of experimental evidence to support the theory of chemical transmission, although much remains to be understood. One of the classical preparations for experiments in this field is the frog sartorious muscle, with its attached nerve. Accordingly, a great deal of the information available at present is related to transmission between efferent motor fibres and skeletal muscle.

When a microelectrode is placed between the nerve fibre and the muscle cell at the point of junction, it can be shown that the axon potential arrives at the junction about 0·8 msec before the potential is set up in the post-junctional tissue. This break in electrical continuity points to some form of non-electrical transmission at the junction. Other experiments indicate that the transmission is almost certainly by the chemical acetylcholine. For example, the addition of eserine to the frog muscle preparation inhibits the enzyme cholinesterase, which hydrolyses acetylcholine. If then the nerve fibre is artificially stimulated, an increasing amount of acetylcholine is released from the end of the fibre. It has also been shown that when acetylcholine is applied by micropipette to the muscle fibre on the precise point of neuromuscular junction, even minute amounts can excite the muscle fibre. When applied elsewhere on the muscle, however, no response is detected.

Less clear results have been obtained in studies of chemical transmission between nerve fibres and tissue such as smooth muscle, glands and cardiac muscle, where the nerves regulate rather than initiate activity. With tissue of this kind no synaptic junctions are made, but the nerve fibres form plexuses within the tissue, the chemical transmitter being released into the surrounding extracellular space. Many smooth muscles are supplied by two sets of nerve fibres, one set releasing acetylcholine and the other noradrenaline. These chemicals oppose each other, one being excitatory and the other inhibitory. Investigations into chemical transmission in this area are further complicated by the action of hormones, which may considerably modify the response of the tissue to nervous stimulation.

At the synaptic junction between two neurones, chemical transmission is known to occur. Direct evidence of this has been obtained from studies of transmission in the peripheral sympathetic ganglia. On stimulation of the preganglionic fibre, acetylcholine is found in the perfusate, and application of acetylcholine to the postganglionic fibre produces stimulation. It is more difficult to obtain evidence for chemical transmission between neurones lying within the central nervous system. Work has been done by introducing acetylcholine iontophoretically through micropipettes, and also by inserting microelectrodes into the brain and spinal cord of the cat. Various substances have been detected in different parts of the brain in different concentrations; these include acetylcholine, noradrenaline, dopamine, histamine, and the prostaglandins. It is generally agreed that these substances and others play some part in synaptic transmission. The prostaglandins, for example, when applied iontophoretically, are seen to stimulate some neurones, but not others. There is still a great deal for us to learn about the chemical nature and the function of most of the transmitters within the central nervous system.

8 Summary and Extension Exercises

I COMPREHENSION EXERCISES

Write out answers to the following questions about the Free Reading passages in Units 1–7.

UNIT 1

(a) Does a weighing machine measure the body as a uniform mass?
(b) Does a weighing machine measure separately the compartments of the body?
(c) What effect has oedema on the total body weight?
(d) If the total body weight remains constant, does this prove that the patient is healthy?
(e) Why is the weighing machine said to be a crude tool?
(f) Is it possible to measure the compartments of the body in any clinic?
(g) How is the size of the cell water calculated?
(h) What experimental techniques are used in the calculation of the size of the bone minerals and the extracellular proteins?

UNIT 2

(a) Where does the process of digestion begin?
(b) What is the function of chewing?
(c) What are the two functions of saliva?
(d) Where do the major processes of digestion occur?
(e) What is the chemical function of the stomach?
(f) What is the physical function of the stomach?
(g) What are lacteals?
(h) Which products of digestion are not absorbed directly into the bloodstream?

UNIT 3

(a) What are the three compartments of the thoracic cavity?
(b) Which is the most important division of the mediastinum, the anterior, posterior, or superior?
(c) How is it that two adjacent layers of serous membrane separate the heart from the fibrous pericardium?
(d) What is the name of the membrane which lines the lungs?
(e) What is the function of the pericardium?
(f) What is the function of the pleura?

UNIT 4

(a) What are the main functions of connective tissue?
(b) What is the main feature of connective tissue?
(c) How are the several types of connective tissue classified?
(d) What kinds of fibres are most commonly found in connective tissue?
(e) Name three kinds of cell commonly found in connective tissue.
(f) Are histiocytes stationary?
(g) Which type of fibre makes up (i) ligaments
                                (ii) tendons
                                (iii) areolar tissue?
(h) In which type of connective tissue is the intercellular matrix hardened by calcium phosphate?

UNIT 5

(a) What are the two major divisions of study in microscopic anatomy?
(b) Can staining reveal invisible structures?
(c) What is meant by basophilia?
(d) Which acid can be traced by the Feulgen Method?
(e) Why is staining said to be selective?
(f) Is it possible to study the living processes of tissue over a period of time, both *in vivo* and *in vitro*?

UNIT 6

(a) What do the results of the two experiments described in paragraph 1 indicate?
(b) What is the function of the sinu-atrial node?
(c) What is the function of the bundle of His?
(d) During the period of diastole, does blood leave the heart?
(e) Is the heart relaxed or contracted during the period of systole?
(f) When does the stroke volume increase?
(g) Why does the left ventricle pump at a higher pressure than the right ventricle?
(h) Do variations in cardiac output depend more on stroke volume than on heart rate?

UNIT 7

(a) The passage discusses the experimental evidence for the chemical transmission of impulses over four main types of junction. The first is the junction between efferent motor fibres and skeletal muscle. What are the other three types of junction mentioned?

(b) For which type of junction do we have most evidence of chemical transmission?

(c) Name two factors which complicate studies of chemical transmission between nerve fibres and smooth muscle.

(d) Name three factors which complicate studies of chemical transmission between two neurones within the central nervous system.

II USE OF LANGUAGE

EXERCISE A *Stating function*

The function of a tissue or organ can be stated in the following ways:
(i) The function of X is *to* + *verb*

EXAMPLE
    The function of the heart is to pump blood.

(ii) X is concerned with *-ing form of verb*

EXAMPLE
    The heart is concerned with pumping blood.

(iii) X acts as *noun*

EXAMPLE
    The heart acts as a pumping-machine.

Change the following sentences so that function is clearly stated. Use the ways of expressing function described above.

EXAMPLE
    Some glands control the metabolic processes.
=   The function of some glands is to control the metabolic processes.

1. The iris adapts the size of the pupil to the amount of light.
2. The bones are a framework for the body.
3. The pleura facilitates the movement of the lungs.
4. The endocrine glands maintain physiological equilibrium.
5. The fat in adipose tissue is an emergency food reserve.

6. Tissue fluid is a 'go-between' between the blood and the cells.
7. The pancreas secretes pancreatic juice and insulin.
8. Bone supports the body.
9. Somatic muscles adapt the individual to the external environment.
10. The muscles of the neck move and support the head.
11. Connective tissue is a supporting matrix for more highly organized structures.
12. Lipase converts fats into fatty acids and glycerol.
13. The muscular walls of the blood vessels regulate the local distribution of blood.
14. The secretion from Brunner's glands protects the lining of the duodenum.

EXERCISE B bring about, provide, facilitate

Write out the following sentences, choosing from the above verbs the appropriate one to fill each blank.

1. The stimulation of the nerve endings ... a reflex emptying of the gall bladder.
2. Saliva ... swallowing.
3. The intercostal muscles ... respiratory movements.
4. The muscles of the hips and thighs ... strength and stability.
5. Loose areolar tissue ... movement between adjacent structures.
6. Progesterone ... a change in the wall of the uterus.
7. The oxidization of food ... heat.
8. A hormone ... the constriction of the gall bladder.
9. Connective tissue ... a supporting matrix for more highly organized structures.
10. The pleura ... two frictionless surfaces which ... the movement of the lungs.
11. The secretion of adrenalin ... a constriction of the arterioles.
12. Dilatation of the blood vessels ... blood flow.
13. Hydrochloric acid ... the medium necessary for the action of pepsin.
14. The superficial fascia ... a surface covering which helps to conserve body heat.
15. The pectoralis major muscle ... the movement of the arm in relation to the trunk.

EXERCISE C aid, assist, help, play an important part

The above expressions are all followed by *in* + noun, or *in* + gerund (*-ing* form of verb):

EXAMPLES
Bile salts assist *in the emulsion* of fats.
Muscular exercise plays an important part *in promoting* good circulation.

help, but NOT the other expressions, may instead be followed by the infinitive (*to* + verb).

EXAMPLE

Subcutaneous fat helps *to protect* underlying organs.

Write out the following sentences, choosing from the expressions above an appropriate one to fill each blank. Add *in* or *to* as necessary.

1. The skin ... the regulation of body temperature.
2. Irregularities of the articular surface ... limiting movement.
3. Striated muscle ... temperature control by generating heat.
4, Ptyalin ... convert starch.
5. Muscular exercise ... promote good circulation.
6. Collagenous tissue ... the repair of injuries.
7. Visceral muscle ... the process of digestion.
8. Bile salts ... emulsifying fats.
9. The abdominal muscles ... respiration and defaecation.
10. Subcutaneous fat ... the protection of underlying organs.

EXERCISE D *Active and passive verbs*

Write out the following sentences, filling in the blanks by choosing the correct form, active or passive, of the verb in brackets at the end of each sentence. Sometimes with a passive verb it may be necessary to add *by*.

EXAMPLES
(a) The cerebral cortex ... all voluntary movement. (regulate)
    The cerebral cortex *regulates* all voluntary movement.
(b) The blood vessels ... along the umbilical cord. (convey)
    The blood vessels *are conveyed* along the umbilical cord.
(c) The teeth of the lower jaw ... the mandibular nerve. (supply)
    The teeth of the lower jaw *are supplied by* the mandibular nerve.

1. The liver ... the amount of glucose in the blood. (regulate)
2. Heat production ... the nervous system. (control)
3. Broken down protoplasm ... into urea, creatinine, or uric acid. (convert)
4. The amniotic cavity ... the foetus. (surround)
5. Mucous membrane ... the cavity of the middle ear. (line)
6. These organs ... fibres from both the sympathetic and the parasympathetic systems. (receive)
7. The vagus nerve ... most of the abdominal viscera. (supply)
8. Cerebro-spinal fluid ... the arachnoid membrane. (secrete)
9. The islets of Langerhans ... insulin. (secrete)
10. The thoracic duct ... lymph from most parts of the body. (drain)
11. The kidneys ... a mass of fat. (surround)

12. The sweat glands ... to secrete at the same time as the blood vessels in the skin ... to dilate. (stimulate)
13. A duct ... the saliva to the mouth. (carry)
14. The lungs ... carbon dioxide and some water. (excrete)
15. Nitrogenous waste ... in the urine. (excrete)
16. Bile ... the liver. (excrete)
17. Enamel ... the crown of each tooth. (cover)
18. The liver ... excess glucose almost as fast as it ... into the blood. (store, absorb)
19. A great number of chemical substances ... during tissue activity. (produce)
20. Fluid ... from the blood into the tissue spaces. (filter)
21. The socket of each tooth ... a layer of fibrous tissue. (line)
22. The blood ... oxygen round the body. (carry)
23. The delicate abdominal organs ... the abdominal muscles. (protect)
24. A pivot joint ... rotation. (allow)
25. Histamine ... dilatation of the capillaries. (bring about)
26. Impulses ... along the vagus and glossopharyngeal nerves to the cardiac centre in the medulla oblongata. (convey)
27. The whole circulatory system ... to meet the needs of the body. (control)
28. The muscular diaphragm of the pelvic floor ... the pelvic organs. (support)
29. Excess carbohydrate ... from the small intestine and ... in the liver. (absorb, store)
30. All proteins ... into amino acids. (convert)
31. The lymph ... bacteria from the tissue spaces. (convey)
32. The lungs ... branches of the vagus nerve. (supply)
33. The phrenic nerve ... the diaphragm. (serve)
34. Muscles ... motor fibres. (activate)
35. The synovial membrane ... foreign particles. (absorb)
36. The thyrotrophic hormone, which ... the pituitary gland, ... the production of thyroxin by the thyroid gland. (secrete, control)

III INFORMATION TRANSFER

Before doing this section look again at Use of Language, Unit 3: Anatomical Terms.

EXERCISE A *Bones: description of shape*

descriptive expressions:

long	U-shaped	with a long shaft
triangular	wedge-shaped	with a slight twist

slender	dagger-shaped	with a rounded head at the proximal end
wide	irregularly-shaped	with a neck and rounded head at the proximal end
curved		with the distal end expanded into two condyles
		with a roller-shaped distal end

Study the above list of descriptive expressions and the following diagrams of bones. Then, picking out suitable expressions, write a sentence describing each bone.

EXAMPLE
The hyoid bone is a U-shaped bone.

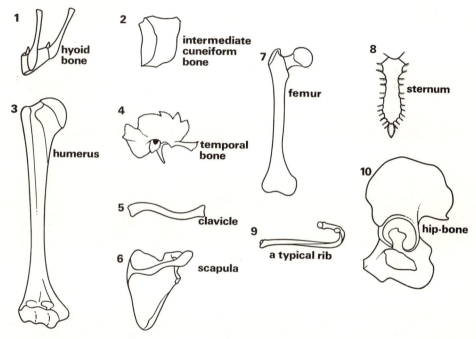

EXERCISE B *Nerves: origin, branches and distribution*

Consult the following table and write descriptions of the nerves in the left-hand column.

EXAMPLES
1. The mental nerve is a branch of the inferior alveolar nerve. It gives off mental and inferior labial branches, which supply the skin of the chin and the lower lip.
2. The great auricular nerve arises from the second and third cervical vertebrae. It emerges from the cervical plexus and gives off anterior and posterior branches. It serves the skin of the side of the head.

TABLE OF NERVES

Name	Origin	Branches	Distribution
1. mental n.	inferior alveolar n.	mental and inferior labial branches	skin of chin and lower lip
2. great auricular n.	C2+C3, cervical plexus	anterior and posterior branches	skin of side of head
3. inferior alveolar n.	mandibular n.	inferior dental and inferior gingival branches, mylohyoid n. and mental n.	teeth and gums of lower jaw, skin of chin and lower lip, mylohyoid muscle, and anterior belly of digastric muscle
4. olfactory n.	olfactory bulb		nasal mucous membrane
5. subclavian n.	C5+C6, brachial plexus		subclavius muscle, sterno-clavicular joint
6. musculo-cutaneous n.	C5–C7, brachial plexus	lateral cutaneous n. of forearm, muscular branches	biceps, brachialis muscles, skin of radial side of forearm
7. masseteric n.	mandibular n.		masseter muscle, temperomandibular joint
8. lateral cutaneous n. of thigh	L2–L3, lumbar plexus		skin of lateral aspect and front of thigh
9. phrenic n.	C3–C5, cervical plexus	pericardial and phrenico-abdominal branches	pericardium, diaphragm
10. greater palatine n.	pterygopalatine ganglion	posterior inferior lateral nasal n.	gums, mucous membrane of soft and hard palates and of inferior concha

EXERCISE C *Muscles: description of action*

1. The following anatomical terms are commonly used in the description of muscle action.

   flexion; to flex (when the angle between the bones is decreased)

   extension; to extend (when the angle between the bones is increased, usually to a more or less straight line) *rotation; to rotate* (when bones are turned one over another, or when the eyeball is turned)

abduction; to abduct (when a limb is moved away from the midline of the body)

adduction; to adduct (when a limb is moved towards the midline of the body)

pronation; to pronate (when the hand is rotated so that the palm is directed posteriorly)

supination; to supinate (when the palm of the hand is rotated to its anatomical position) (see Unit 3)

inversion; to invert (when the sole of the foot is rotated towards the midline of the body)

eversion; to evert (when the sole of the foot is rotated away from the midline of the body)

dorsiflexion; to dorsiflex (when the foot is pulled up in front of the leg)

plantarflexion; to plantarflex (when the foot is pointed downwards)

State what action is shown in each of the following diagrams.

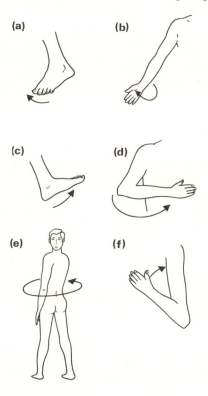

2. Write brief descriptions of the motor units presented in the following table.

EXAMPLE

The brachialis muscle, which flexes the forearm, arises from the anterior aspect of the humerus and is inserted into the coronoid process of the ulna. It is supplied by the musculocutaneous and the radial nerves.

Name	Origin	Insertion	Innervation	Action
1. m. brachialis	anterior aspect of humerus	coronoid process of ulna	musculo-cutaneous, radial nn.	flexes forearm
2. m. anconeus	back of lateral epicondyle of humerus	olecranon and posterior surface of ulna	radial n.	extends forearm
3. m. crico-arytenoideus lateralis	arch of cricoid cartilage	muscular process of arytenoid cartilage	recurrent laryngeal n.	approximates vocal folds
4. m. peroneus brevis	lateral surface of fibula	tuberosity of fifth metatarsal bone	superficial peroneal n.	everts foot
5. m. extensor pollicis longus	posterior surface of ulna and interosseous membrane	back of distal phalanx of thumb	posterior interosseous n.	extends, adducts thumb
6. m. rectus superior bulbi	common tendinous ring	sclera	oculomotor n.	adducts, raises, rotates eyeball medially
7. m. rectus femoris	anterior inferior iliac spine, rim of acetabulum	base of patella, tuberosity of tibia	femoral n.	extends leg, flexes thigh
8. m. semi-tendinosus	tuberosity of ischium	upper part of medial surface of tibia	sciatic n.	flexes and rotates leg medially, extends thigh
9. m. splenius cervicis	spinous processes of upper thoracic vertebrae	transverse processes of upper cervical vertebrae	cervical n.	extends, rotates head and neck
10. m. pronator quadratus	anterior surface and border of ulna	anterior surface and border of radius	anterior interosseous n.	pronates forearm

EXERCISE D *Arteries: the aorta and its branches*

(a) Copy the diagram below into your notebook. Read the following passage and complete the labelling of the diagram, using the italicized words in the passage.

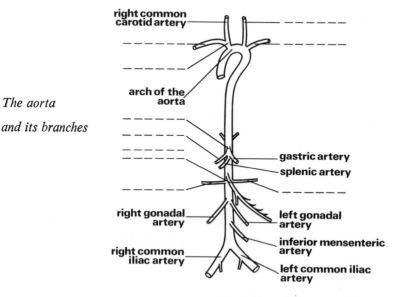

The aorta

and its branches

The aortic arch gives off on the right the *innominate artery*, which after two inches divides into the *right subclavian artery* and the right common carotid. Then, on the left side of the arch, the aorta gives off first the *left common carotid artery* and then the *left subclavian artery*.

The aorta then passes down through the thorax into the abdomen, where it gives off several branches. The most important of these are the *coeliac artery,* which divides into three branches: the gastric artery, the splenic artery, and the *hepatic artery*. About 1 cm inferior to the coeliac artery the *superior mesenteric artery* is given off, and immediately below this the *right and left renal arteries* arise.

(b) Complete the passage, referring to the diagram.

EXERCISE E *Veins: the hepatic portal system*

(a) Study the following table and write out the completed sentences.

TABLE OF VEINS

vein	receives blood from	drains into
superior mesenteric v.	capillaries in the small intestine and the ascending and transverse colon	portal v.
splenic v.	capillaries in the spleen	portal v.
inferior mesenteric v.	posterior part of large intestine	splenic v.
right and left gastric vv.	the stomach	portal v.
portal v.	superior mesenteric v. splenic v. right and left gastric vv.	capillaries in the liver

1. The capillaries in the small intestine and the ascending and transverse colon unite to form the ......
2. The superior mesenteric vein ...... the portal vein.
3. The inferior mesenteric vein ...... the splenic vein.
4. The splenic vein receives blood from ......
5. ...... receives blood from the inferior mesenteric vein.
6. The capillaries in the liver ...... the portal vein.
7. The superior mesenteric vein, the splenic vein, and the right and left gastric veins join to form the ......
8. The inferior mesenteric vein receives blood from the ......

(b) Copy the following diagram and complete the labelling using the information in section (a). Write out the paragraph below, filling in the blanks with reference to the diagram.

The hepatic portal system

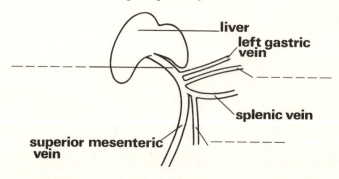

The capillaries in the small intestine and the ascending and transverse colon unite to form the ...... The capillaries in the spleen join to form the ...... This ...... the inferior mesenteric vein, which drains blood from the posterior part of ...... The superior mesenteric vein and the ...... join to form the ...... It receives blood from the ...... and then drains ......

IV ESSAY WRITING

Write a short essay based on the following notes. Combine the sentences in any way you wish, changing the grammatical patterns if necessary. Divide your essay into paragraphs and give the essay a title.

the term 'homeostasis' was introduced by Cannon in 1929
it describes the physiological equilibrium of living organisms
the word is derived from Greek
it means a 'state of sameness'
this does not mean an immobile fixed state
it may vary
it remains relatively constant
the concept was largely anticipated by Claude Bernard
Claude Bernard was a famous French physiologist
he first put forward the view that the human body is a self-regulating system
he said that the body is protected from changes in the external environment
he said that it is protected by the 'milieu interieur'
the 'milieu interieur' consists of the extracellular fluid in the blood and lymph
every cell of the body is bathed in this fluid
it constitutes an internal, or local, environment for all the body cells
the principal function of the organs of the body is to maintain homeostasis
the kidney regulates the osmotic pressure
the action of the lungs ensures a fairly constant level of oxygen
the subcutaneous blood vessels dilate when the body is over-heated
this allows for increased evaporation
the blood sugar concentration is held fairly steady by the liver
the muscles help to regulate the physico-chemical state of the internal environment both directly and indirectly
cardiac muscle regulates it directly
cardiac muscle pumps blood
the muscles of posture and movement affect it directly
they help to defend the body against the external environment
they help to bring it food
every tissue in the body plays a part in the maintenance of homeostasis
the nervous system and the secretory glands control the tissues of the body
a certain type of control system brings about homeostasis

it is known as a servo-system
a servo-system is basically a control system which includes a closed loop
the closed loop may also be called feedback
the flexion reflex is a simple instance of a servo-system at work
the flexion reflex occurs when e.g. the foot receives a painful stimulus
the foot is withdrawn by flexion of the leg
the foot is the receptor
the central nervous system is the adjustor
the leg muscle is the effector
the receptor affects the adjustor
the adjustor controls the effector
this constitutes a reflex arc
the effector moderates the receptor
it removes the painful stimulus from the receptor
thus a closed loop is formed in the control system
all control systems effecting homeostasis are systems of this type
usually they are more complex
obviously, effector organs need not be muscle
the pancreas is an effector organ in its secretion of insulin
insulin is necessary for the conversion of sugar
the receptor organ might be e.g. the olefactory bulb
the adjustor may be one of various kinds of signal
these are physico-chemical, thermal, electrical, etc.
signals are usually transmitted by nerve impulses
at the synapses they are transmitted chemically
certain signals may be transmitted hormonally
much research has been devoted to the study of the control systems of the
     body
a great deal more research will be necessary
many difficulties face the researcher
experimental techniques may distort the control system under study
e.g. in the flexion reflex one experimental technique is to apply electrical
     stimulation to a sensory fibre in the leg
this brings about flexion of the leg
this brings about withdrawal of the foot
under these experimental conditions, the response of withdrawal has no
     effect on the initiating stimulation
the effector does not moderate the receptor
there is no closed loop
the closed loop is an essential feature of the control system under study
other difficulties face the researcher
these may be due to the complexity of the control systems themselves
e.g. in the regulation of the ventilation of the lungs, a suitable rate of blood
     flow is brought about by a number of control systems
these control systems interact.